The year 1977 brought the first of the skin problems. Sensitive skin runs in Dan's family and we were not overly concerned. The days of roadbuilding in the Nevada desert came to mind for prolonged exposure to the sun and its subsequent damage, but with age had come wisdom and for years he had worn a cap or hat when playing golf or during any extended period out-of-doors. In March, actinic keratoses (precancerous lesions) were removed from his face and arms. More were removed in April and in August. He then started wearing long-sleeved shirts and was even more cautious to protect his skin from the sun's rays. These skin problems continued through 1978, but all areas were benign and were successfully treated.

As I put these events in chronological order in preparation for writing this book, I wonder just how much one episode may have related to the next. What combination of events led up to the traumatic experience which awaited us? How much can the immune system withstand? Should we have known—right from the beginning? From the first diagnosis? Perhaps we did, but we kept our doubts pushed aside. We lived one day at a time. Perhaps, after all, that is what made it bearable and enabled us to make the maximum use and to squeeze the maximum happiness from the time which we were to be given.

DIARY OF COURAGE

Coping with Life-threatening Illness

Mary Woodward Priest

Strawberry Hill Press

Copyright © 1990 by Mary Woodward Priest

Strawberry Hill Press
2594 15th Avenue
San Francisco, California 94127

Edited by Anne M. Ingram

Proofread by Catherine J. Nichols

Front cover photo of Daniel Hillman Goodrich Priest by Mary Woodward Priest; back cover photo of Mary Woodward Priest by Vastine Studio, Inc. of Santa Rosa, California

Cover by Ku, Fu-sheng

Typeset and designed by Cragmont Publications, Oakland, California

Printed by Edwards Brothers, Inc., Lillington, North Carolina

Manufactured in the United States of America

Library of Congress Cataloging-in-Publication Data

Priest, Mary Woodward.
    Diary of courage : coping with life-threatening illness /Mary Woodward Priest.
        p.   cm.
    Includes bibliographical references (p.   )
    ISBN 0-89407-099-1 : $9.95
        1. Priest, Daniel Hillman Goodrich—Health. 2. Prostate—Cancer—Patients—California—Biography. 3. Critically ill. 4. Adjustment (Psychology)
I. Title.
RC280.P7P644   1990
362.1'9699463'0092—dc20   90-9502
[B]   CIP

Dedication

In loving memory of my husband, Daniel Hillman Goodrich Priest, who shared with me twenty-nine beautiful years. Though his life span fell far short of the Biblical three score and ten, his Christian influence upon the lives of his family, his friends and his colleagues will continue long after his death.

Table of Contents

Preface

BEFORE MY HUSBAND DAN lost his battle with prostate cancer he said to me, "Mary, when this is over, you must write our story. You're a professional writer. You can do it. No one else can. Reading of our experiences will be helpful to those who will come after us."

The American Cancer Society estimates that in 1990 about 1,010,000 people will be diagnosed as having cancer, that it will strike three out of ten Americans living today and enter the lives of three out of every four American families. During this year there will be about 502,000 deaths from the disease. No one as yet knows why some cancers stop or go into remission and why some continue to travel.

The lessons we learned are equally applicable to any life-threatening illness.

When Dan received his original diagnosis, we were prepared by our faith in God, our love for each other and his personal courage to meet the spiritual, emotional and physical demands of coping with this dread disease. We did not realize, however, the depths to which our faith and courage would be tested; the feelings of inadequacy, even guilt which would arise and then be offset by the sheer joy of living. Nor were we prepared for the changes which have occurred in the medical-care delivery system in recent years and the effects of these changes on the patient and the patient's family.

I was born and raised on a farm in central Illinois; Dan in Carson City, Nevada, when it was still a small town. We had been treated, when necessary, by old-fashioned family doctors who ministered not only to the patient but to the whole family. During the early years of our marriage in the mid-1950s, we lived in the San Francisco Bay Area and were fortunate to have attending physicians who carried on this tradition.

During the diagnosis and treatment of Dan's illness, we became involved in the referral service which took us from specialist to specialist, each different, each a total stranger, each requiring an adjustment on the part of the patient as Dan encountered new methods of treatment, new opinions. Naturally, each specialist was primarily interested in his own area of expertise; but, more importantly, they did not know Dan. They did not know he was a person who could bear a lot of pain, who never complained until pain was almost unendurable; a person who kept his calm in any emergency and who stoically coped with whatever life had to offer.

Dealing with so many people we did not know and who did not know us gave us a feeling of loss of control over our lives. We felt that Dan was being regarded as a collection of unrelated parts instead of a whole person. We were sometimes confused; our questions went unanswered. We were even doubtful as to which doctor we should call when an emergency arose.

The hospital system was equally baffling. We had been exposed to convalescent hospitals in the search for proper care of Dan's elderly mother, a stroke victim, but we had no idea we would even have to consider such a facility for him. It was unthinkable to us given his age and his illness. We had to learn the restrictions of the acute care hospitals, the convalescent hospitals and had to consider hospice and out-patient care.

We thought we had been meticulous in keeping our personal financial affairs in order but discovered that we had overlooked important changes.

As we encountered each new obstacle and faced each new problem, we wanted to turn our disappointments and frustrations into something positive. We became convinced that others could benefit from the knowledge we had gained. We were making our way through the greatest challenge of our lives. We felt it would be a comfort to those who follow to know that they were not alone, that others had traveled the same path before them, and that in reading of our experiences they would find information and inspiration which would be of help to them. This became our dream: That our story would provide not only helpful information but also inspiration that people can and do face these traumatic events without losing quality of life and that regardless of the physical outcome, the human spirit does, indeed, triumph.

Since my husband's death, I've talked with many friends and acquaintances who face similar situations. They have asked questions which are answered in this book. I am more convinced than ever that Dan's wishes for such a book were wise. This conviction has given me the courage to present our story.

While other books have been written on the subject of cancer, they tend to be specialized, to present only a limited view of the illness. *Diary of Courage*, this one slim volume, treats it all.

Part 1 is a diary of the most important dates in the two-year drama, connected by narrative. It illustrates the effects of the disease on the lives of average people, the reactions of friends, the challenges of dealing with the medical community, sources of support, and the courage and faith of the patient.

Part 2, based upon the events of Part 1, is a guide, a "how-to," filled with information and ideas for coping with the moods of the patient, the specialization of doctors and hospitals, practical tips on patient care and how to preplan to alleviate the burdens of such times.

It is my hope that what we learned and what I have continued to learn in my ongoing search for knowledge and understanding will be helpful to the reader. Dan's request that I write our story was his final gift to me. This book is our gift to the reader.

Introduction

SOME TIME IN THE PAST, this story has its beginning. We just don't know when that beginning was and we were never to find out.

It could have been as early as 1925 when a round, happy, healthy blue-eyed baby boy underwent his first surgery. Doctors said it was a thyroglossal cyst. Dan was only two at the time.

Aunt Sophie recalls, "The trouble came on quite suddenly. Dan made a noise. Kind of like air passing through somewhere. It was not so much that he was having trouble breathing, but the strange, gurgling noise that he made was what caused the alarm. The doctor operated right away and the baby seemed fine after about two weeks."

The only visible reminder of that surgery was a small scar around Dan's throat; yet the glandular system affects so many functions of the body and is especially important for growth and metabolism. Did some developmental abnormality later signal the growth of cancerous cells?

We can look back to the years 1939 and 1940 when Dan spent his summer vacations from high school working as a caddie at Glenbrook Lodge on the California-Nevada border where he spent his days under the hot mountain sun. During his limited leisure time, he was also out-of-doors playing tennis. We now know that ultraviolet rays from the sun cause injury to unprotected skin, causing more work for the body's machinery for fighting illness—the immune system.

Maybe it began in 1942 when his time away from the Occidental College (California) campus found him employed as a chainman on a road construction survey crew for the State of Nevada. I can visualize him now—stripped to the waist, bare of head, slim hips encased in tight-fitting Levis tucked into high-laced boots, protection from the hundreds of rattlers the crew killed for each mile of road, and simmering under temperatures of one-hundred-forty degrees in the blazing desert sun of Battle Mountain, Nevada. Forty years later he was treated for actinic keratoses, pre-cancerous lesions related to overexposure to the sun.

Perhaps the story's roots lie during the years July 1943 to August 1946, when Dan served in the Navy during World War II. An outstanding student, Dan had received the Bausch & Lomb Honorary Science Award, the American Legion Patriotic Essay Award and the American Legion Scholarship Award during his years at Carson High School, Carson City, Nevada. He enlisted in the Navy V-12 Program at Occidental College, California, and was called to active duty July 1, 1943. He was sent to Pre-Midshipmen's School at Asbury Park, New Jersey; Midshipmen's School at Notre Dame, Indiana; Naval Training School (Pre-Radar) at Bowdoin College, Maine; and, finally, the Naval Training School (Radar) at Massachusetts Institute of Technology, Boston. His specialty was radio, radar and sonar, and when he received his commission as Lieutenant, j.g., he was qualified as Group Radar Officer, Division Officer and Radio Materiel Officer. He served as Electronic Technical Officer aboard the USS Achelous and the USS Samuel N. Moore in the Asiatic-Pacific Theatre after additional training at the Fleet Training Center, Oahu. Near the end of his tour of duty, he spent three months in the China seas with stops at Manila and Shanghai, but most of that time he was in Tsingtao, China. He was separated from service at San Francisco in August 1946 and returned to school, transferring to the University of California at Berkeley to study business and insurance.

What were the hazards associated with that early radar and sonar equipment? When x-rays first came into use, they were considered such a valuable aid to medicine that they were used in a totally indiscriminate manner. They were a part of every annual physical and every semi-annual visit to the dentist. They were even used to check the fit of children's shoes. Now we know their dangers.

Could it have been in 1954? It was our first year of marriage, and for our vacation we had planned to drive to Illinois to meet my family. Dan started the trip with a slight cold, but the second day out, he was burning with fever and experiencing drenching sweats. A doctor in Salt Lake City, Utah gave him a shot of penicillin and some medication and told him to stay in bed. A couple of days later, the fever was down, the sweats had stopped and we resumed our journey. During his struggle with cancer, however, I learned to associate drenching sweats with the times the cancer was most active.

The following day we were involved in an auto accident near Rawlins, Wyoming and Dan suffered a spontaneous pneumothorax. After a week of bedrest, he was released with instructions not to lift anything heavy or engage in any strenuous activity. When we returned to our home in Berkeley and Dan checked in with his personal physician, his lung was normal.

It was in 1958 that Dan suddenly lost the central vision in his right eye, his sense of taste, and he had some difficulty in muscular coordination. His handwriting at the time was barely legible. His speech was slightly slurred. Was it stress? His father had suffered a serious heart attack. I had had major surgery. He was involved in a job change at work. This strange physical phenomenon remained unexplained, even after an electroencephalogram and two spinal taps. A possible diagnosis, which caused us great mental anguish for years, was multiple sclerosis. However, all the symptoms were temporary and cleared up within a few months, except for the central vision in his right eye, which never returned.

In 1959 his doctor discovered an iron deficiency and gave him potent iron shots for a number of weeks.

In 1960 we bought our first home, newly built on one-third acre of bare dirt. From then on, we were homeowners, involved in landscaping and lawn maintenance, and Dan liberally used chlordane, DDT, 2, 4–D, malathion, dalapon and miscellaneous chemicals to control weeds and pests. Since then, many of these same chemicals have been banned or restricted. What damage might they have already done?

In spite of these episodes, during most of our married life, Dan was healthy, active, almost tireless and a man who enjoyed life to the fullest. He studied at night and earned his Chartered Property and Casualty Underwriter Degree, served as deacon in our church, and together we worked as superintendents of the junior department, participated in membership drives and finance campaigns. He continued his participation in Alpha Tau Omega activities, a fraternity he had joined in 1941 in college, and added an interest in lodge work, becoming a member of the Grand Lodge, Free and Accepted Masons of the State of California.

After our move to Santa Rosa, California in 1963, Dan went for several years without seeing a physician except for the annual office physical. It was in 1973 that the x-rays, which were a part of this annual checkup, revealed a spot on his lung. In March of that year, he underwent surgery, *Bronchoscopy with Right Middle Lobectomy*, for removal of a collection of tissue which was benign and the sort of growth, we were informed, commonly found in persons who have lived in the desert. However, this was the same lung which had been involved in the spontaneous pneumothorax almost twenty years earlier.

At the end of six months, the cardiologist who had performed the surgery gave Dan a clean bill of health. I then resigned my position after a thirty-year career in life insurance office management, and on December 30, 1973, we were off to Carmel to attend the Bing Crosby Golf Tournament. We had just checked into our motel when Dan developed a high fever. His body was hot and sweat poured from him, drenching the bed. Was it just a "bug"?

In May 1975 Dan visited a local family physician for a complete examination. He was just six weeks short of his fifty-second birthday.

"For men over fifty, rectal examinations should be a routine part of every physical checkup—done by a doctor whose finger is expertly sensitized in the detection of early prostatic disorders." *Our Human Body*, published in 1962 by the Reader's Digest Association, Inc., page 315. Now, over twenty-five years later, the American Cancer Society recommends that "every man over 40 should have a rectal examination as part of his regular annual physical checkup." Their statistics tell us that prostate cancer is the third leading cause of cancer deaths in men in the United States. Yet none of Dan's physical examinations ever included a rectal examination.

Though the local doctor was not as thorough as his doctor in the Bay Area, Dan did not think to question this. He had no symptoms and felt fine. After the 1973 surgery, he had quit smoking and had gained weight, but during 1976 he dieted and got his weight down to excellent standards.

The year 1977 brought the first of the skin problems. Sensitive skin runs in Dan's family and we were not overly concerned. The days of road-building in the Nevada desert came to mind for Dan's prolonged exposure to the sun and its subsequent damage, but with age had come wisdom and for years he had worn a cap or hat when playing golf or during any extended period out-of-doors. In March, actinic keratoses (precancerous lesions) were removed from his face and arms. More were removed in April and in August. He then started wearing long-sleeved shirts and was even more cautious to protect his skin from the sun's rays. These skin problems continued through 1978 but all areas were benign and were successfully treated.

As I put these events in chronological order in preparation for writing this book, I wonder just how much one episode may have

related to the next. What combination of events led up to the traumatic experience which awaited us? How much can the immune
system withstand? Should we have known—right from the beginning? From the first diagnosis? Perhaps we did, but we kept our
doubts pushed aside. We lived one day at a time. Perhaps, after all,
that is what made it bearable and enabled us to make the maximum
use and to squeeze the maximum happiness from the time which we
were to be given.

Prologue

THE YEAR OF 1980 began with great promise. We were both in good health. Our entire medical expense of 1979 had consisted of two visits each to the dentist and one to the ophthalmologist. We attended church at 11:30 P.M. on New Year's Eve, December 31, 1979, to renew our vows in the manner of John Wesley and his Methodist Church and returned home to toast the new year, as had become our custom. We no longer enjoyed the expensive dinner dances and long nights of celebrations that had marked our earlier years. Like attending church each Sunday, which started the week in a positive vein, the New Year's Eve service began the year with a rededication to the Christian principles by which we tried to live.

Dan was now Past Master of his Masonic Blue Lodge. He had spent a number of years breathing new life into an almost dying chapter, bringing in the energy and enthusiasm of friends and colleagues his own age. It was under his direction that he and the other officers had memorized the beautiful Masonic Funeral Service which they were called upon to perform frequently. He also continued his participation in coaching new candidates for their degrees. He was soon to be installed as King of the Royal Arch Masons.

Dan was treasurer of the camera club and I was editor of the club bulletin. Photography was a more recent interest of Dan's but one he had taken up with great verve, spending weekends taking courses at Mendocino Art Center. We both loved travel and, as he was looking forward to an early retirement, possibly at age sixty-two, our plan was that he would take pictures and I would write text for travel features. We had already sold a number of our articles and photos of trips to Canada, Europe and England to various newspapers and magazines. He had already selected the type of small self-contained camper we would buy for our further wanderings when the time came. He had even started to collect supplies for the dark room he planned to build.

In January, we were looking forward to a visit from my mother, to celebrate her eightieth birthday. Mother's health was becoming increasingly delicate from her progressive heart disease, and we looked forward to this, what we all knew would be her last, visit to California. She was to arrive on January 9.

Part I—The Diary

(Coping with Life-threatening Illness)

Phase 1: Cancer!

July 26, 1980

Dan stood at the edge of the crowd which awaited the arrival of the Trans World Airlines flight from Denver. It was 8:30 P.M.. As I searched the expectant faces I felt a twinge of disappointment that he was standing so far away. I ran toward him as fast as my own tired body, burdened with heavy purse, camera and fifteen pounds of carry-on luggage would allow.

The Soroptimist Federation Convention had been exhausting. As newly-installed president of the Santa Rosa club, I was an official delegate and I had attended long days of meetings, followed by late night sessions, banquets and entertainment. There had been too much food, too much drink and too much excitement. Denver's altitude and midsummer heat had prevented me from sleeping when I did get to bed. As a perfect climax to such a fatiguing time, my seatmates on the flight home were two small boys traveling alone, both of whom were sick on the plane. So much for catching forty winks en route. I collapsed into Dan's arms. My first words to him were, "What did the doctor say?"

He also looked tired. I remembered what his mother had told me about his beautiful blue eyes. "His grandfather always said they would break some girl's heart someday." Tonight they did make me feel sad because they were unusually serious. I was scared. I didn't know why.

He replied, "We'll talk later—when we're back at the car."

We started the long walk through the terminal and I noted that his limp had worsened during the week I had been away. Or was it just more noticeable to me? I stood quietly and anxiously within the circle of his arms as we waited for my luggage.

The pain in Dan's groin had started a few months earlier. A muscle pull, we thought. The winter had been wet, and he'd been confined to office work during the week. But, avid golfer that he was, he was a faithful Saturday morning visitor to the country club where he played with his regular foursome, "The Dawn Patrol." They were on the course as soon as the thaw of the frost allowed, unless rain was pouring down. Frequently the course was wet, the grass deep and slippery and a physical strain to walk through, even without carrying a bag of heavy clubs. Dan had played each Saturday possible, come home and taken some aspirins, soaked in a hot tub and rested up until the following week. Now the course is dry, the walking easy, but the pain has persisted.

His first visit to his physician resulted in a diagnosis of arthritis, but he had a more complete physical and additional tests during the week I was away. We had visited briefly on the phone and he again mentioned the arthritis, adding that we would talk more when I got home. As we made our way through the labyrinth of the garage, I waited to hear what he had learned. The results of all those tests.

We walked for a long time. Suddenly, I realized Dan had forgotten where he had parked the car. An overwhelming coldness of fear ran through my body. Dan never lost his sense of direction. His memory was almost photographic and his concentration was such that he could watch TV, read a magazine and listen to my chatter and absorb it all.

"Which car did you bring?" I asked, knowing full well I would have recognized either.

"Liz," he replied. Liz. Our 1964 Dodge convertible which he loved. We had special-ordered it from Detroit and it had long since passed the 100,000-mile mark. Every summer the top came down on Memorial Day weekend and went back up only after daylight saving time ended. He drove it to work every day, Panama straw hat shading his eyes and occasionally keeping the foggy drizzle off his glasses.

We finally located the sporty brown car with its black top and loaded the luggage into the trunk. Dan paid the parking fee and edged out into the traffic of 101 Freeway North, headed home. Only then did he begin to talk.

"The doctor thinks it could be a disease of the bone, Paget's Disease."

"What can be done about it?" I kept my eyes on the road and tried to make my voice lighter than I felt. I was not familiar with the term.

"He says they have various methods of keeping one comfortable, but there is no cure."

I thought of my sister's continuing battle with arthritis. There was no cure for that either but it seemed to progress more slowly and at least I was familiar with it.

"There is another possibility," Dan continued. "Prostate cancer."

Cancer! The word struck terror into me. For a moment I was completely numb. I thought of my father. He had lost his battle with cancer when he was only fifty-six. I tried to push the thought aside. That was nearly thirty years ago. Now I read of the great strides made in cancer treatment—the improved cure rate. I did not dare trust my voice, but Dan seemed not to notice.

He added, "I have appointments for a bone scan on Monday and with a urologist on Wednesday."

I had to say something. "We'll just have to wait and see what these additional tests reveal. Perhaps all these possibilities are wrong and we'll have nothing to worry about." But my voice sounded strained, even to me.

As we drove on, we caught up on each other's activities during the week we had been apart, but periodically we lapsed into silence, each lost in his own thoughts. What was Dan feeling? Was he as frightened as I?

I tried to calm the panic I felt inside. All the death claim files I had reviewed and approved for payment during my days in life insurance came to mind. The word cancer appeared in so many of them. It was the second leading cause of death after heart disease. I chanted a simple, continuous prayer. *Please, God, let it be anything but cancer.*

I studied Dan's face. He was so strong, so young-looking, so virile. *No. It's unthinkable. There has to be some mistake, some other explanation.* I reached over and clasped his hand. "Whatever it is, we'll lick it!"

He slipped his arm around my shoulder and as I snuggled closer, he said firmly, "Of course we will."

July 30, 1980

I waited anxiously for Dan's return from his 3 P.M. appointment with the urologist. He had his bone scan on Monday and on the way home got a prescription filled for aspirin with codeine, his first pain medication. Today we should learn the worst—or the best. Dan seemed a bit subdued. I mixed a drink and we sat down to talk.

"The urologist feels that the likelihood is the cancer." He took a sip of his drink.

I felt the color drain from my face and said nothing.

"He wants to do surgery. He talked about treatment with hormones and their side effects and he recommends that, in my case, surgery would be the best course of action to take."

Again I waited.

"The doctor says it is the male hormone that feeds this kind of cancer," he explained, "and he recommends removing both testicles so that no more of the hormone will be produced."

"I see."

I tried to assimilate this new and shocking information. Dan just turned fifty-seven, though he looks and acts much younger. I'm fifty-four. Hardly ages when one looks forward to a life of celibacy. The most important consideration, however, is Dan's life, his well-being. I wonder how he will cope with the loss of his manhood, should that occur. What effect it might have on our relationship. I find comfort in the knowledge that Dan has always known who he is. He possesses a depth of character and self-confidence that enables him to meet life's disappointments. If anyone can accept such a crushing blow, I'm certain it will be he. Can I cope, too? *I have to*!

I smiled at him with what I hoped was reassurance. "Honey, if the surgery will stop the cancer and save your life, there's really no question, is there?"

"No, I guess not. The urologist wants us to think about it, talk it over with my family physician and then let him know."

We prayed and pushed the negative thoughts aside.

Now Dan waits and though his manner is calm, I note that as he sits in his chair perusing his *Business Week*, he sometimes has a faraway look. He, too, is pondering his fate.

August 10, 1980

At my insistence, after church we drove to San Francisco to see a Kachina Doll exhibit in Golden Gate Park. In one of my bitchier moments, I prodded Dan into going. "If you can play golf on Saturday, surely you can do something with me on Sunday."

Already, I am fearful of missing his company. He has always had so much energy. Enough to pursue his own interests without neglecting the activities we share. Now this seems to be coming to a close. I grab for every moment!

We took our cameras along, carefully hidden in the trunk of the car, but as we got out, Dan decided to change lenses. He removed his camera bag from the trunk, made the switch and left the remaining items on the floor of the car. When we returned an hour later, the window of the car had been smashed and everything stolen. A man who lived nearby came to our aid with a brush and towels and helped us clean up the mess of broken glass. Then we stopped at park police headquarters to make our report. I was so shaken I was almost in tears and wanted to drive straight home, but Dan refused to let the events spoil our day. We stopped at Tiburon for dinner as planned. I know he was in pain, but he refused to let it, or the robbery, ruin our outing. I'm so ashamed that I ask so much of him.

August 15, 1980

After work today, I met Dan at the urologist's office for our conference. It was my first introduction to this new doctor. A small man with cold, impassive blue eyes hiding behind steel-rimmed glasses and wearing a bow tie gave me a nod of recognition and a curt "Hello."

Dan placed a long distance call to his former physician in Berkeley and talked with him briefly. Then the two doctors conversed. Surgery was the treatment recommended by both.

I sat silent and still, watching the scene unfold before my eyes, studying this new specialist who had entered our lives so dramatically and whose aloof, clinical manner removed him totally from the bombshell he had dropped upon us. Gathering courage, I asked him, "What will such an operation do to marital relations?"

He looked at me as if I were totally stupid. Perhaps the question was, but as private as Dan and I are in such matters, I still wanted verification.

"Well, I should think it would end it," he replied, and somewhat impatiently waited for our decision.

For days we have pondered about this. We have both experienced many disappointments in life. The anticipated children which never arrived. The loss of much-loved fathers. Frustrations in our careers. This, then, is to be one more. Our faith has seen us through the others. It will have to sustain us through this, too. The surgery is to be done next Wednesday.

August 20, 1980

We arrived at the hospital at 7:30 A.M. Dan was out late last night, enjoying his Past Masters' Night at lodge. Neither of us slept well. In silence we took care of the paperwork at the admissions desk. There is always such a sense of dread as one signs those permission forms with their chilling warnings. I have signed several such forms for myself in the past. Somehow it is more ominous putting Dan's life into the surgeon's hands. I feel so helpless.

Formalities completed, we were ushered into a dingy, four-bed ward filled with noisy, elderly, unshaved men, shuffling around through air blue with cigarette smoke. It looked more like an old folks' home than a hospital. Dan did not seem bothered by it, but when they started prepping him, I went to the desk to see about another room. None was available. Perhaps a two-bed room would open up later. I fervently hoped so and was disappointed that the urologist, who was to perform the surgery, had not arranged for more suitable accommodations.

Returning to the ward, I pulled the curtain to give us some privacy and we joked together as Dan dressed in the leggings, cap and other strange clothing that one dons for the operating room. All too soon, I was walking alongside the gurney, holding his hand and giving him one last quick kiss. Everything was going to be okay. Then he was out of sight behind those forbidding, swinging doors.

The waiting room was full of people. Waiting rooms always are as the drama of human existence unfolds daily in such surroundings. A television set brightened one corner but attracted viewers only for a few minutes at a time. The background noise, however, relieved a bit of the tension which gripped the room. Some folks made trips to the coffee machine. Most sat quietly, lost in thought.

I sank into a corner of a couch, picked up a book and tried to read. After several pages, I realized I did not remember a single word. I started over, but my mind continued to stray. In just a few short weeks, our world has been turned upside-down. On the surface we have continued as usual—work, golf, attending our regular meetings, mowing lawns, swimming in the pool. Each Sunday we are in our pew at church where I pray for Dan's recovery, for wisdom to keep him safe and happy and for strength to never let him down as he faces this trying time.

My thoughts are a continuous prayer. As I talk with God, I

remember my father and his surgery. His was not successful. Dan's has to be.

Some time later, the surgeon came out of the operating room and sat down beside me. They had tested tissue in three areas, only one of which appeared to be malignant. I was immediately encouraged, but the elation did not last.

"I still think we should proceed with the complete surgery now," he said. "It will save Dan another anesthetic and there is nothing to be gained by waiting. Mrs. Priest, I would like your permission to go ahead."

He exuded no warmth, compassion, or understanding. He simply wanted my permission. Dan's manhood, perhaps even his very life, was now in my hands. I felt suffocated. My God, what a decision! I was not prepared for this.

The doctor continued, "Of course, it's entirely up to you, but I feel the sooner done the better."

Here was what we had agonized over. We had prayed about it. We had decided that if such drastic measures were required, they would be taken. Yet the odds were different now. Only one of the three areas tested was malignant. I knew such tests were not infallible. Could even that have been a mistake? Could there be some other reason for Dan's pain? Why not remove only the suspect area and leave all else intact?

He explained again that the male hormone testosterone fed the cancer and that the chances for Dan's complete recovery would be better if such production was stopped. He waited, somewhat impatiently.

I took a deep breath and told him to go ahead, fervently praying that if he had had the opportunity, Dan would have made the same decision.

The doctor returned to the operating room. I returned to my book, swallowing hard to hold back the tears; but when the hospital chaplain came over and said, "I understand you have troubles," the tears burst through. I went into her office where I cried, almost hysterically, for several minutes.

When the doctor came in later, I was glad that I was in better control. He gave me no feeling of solace or even any encouragement.

"We will just have to wait and see what the surgery accomplishes," were his only words.

I knew Dan would soon be taken from the recovery room, so I went into the bathroom, splashed cold water on my face and tried to regain my composure. It was not long until the gurney passed by and I accompanied it down the corridor.

Then we were settled into a two-bed room and even the second bed was empty. Thank heavens we were to have a little privacy.

By the time Dan awakened, I had regained my composure. He smiled and looked up at me inquiringly. Smiling back, I nodded yes, then said, "It's okay. The surgery will do the job. We'll still lick it."

He seemed content and went back to sleep.

Toward evening, Dan became fully awake in time to talk with the surgeon about the operation.

"Cystoscopy, Needle Biopsy Prostate, Bilateral Simple Orchiectomy." The findings, *"Carcinoma of Prostate with Metastases."* The operation was a simple one and he said that Dan could go home the next day. He inquired if there was any pain.

"No," Dan replied.

"That," said the surgeon, "is a very good sign."

It is the first good news he has brought us. Dan and I hugged each other. We've won our battle! I came home in high spirits and slept well.

August 22, 1980

We spent the day reading and sorting through photographs. This evening Dan suddenly developed a very high fever. All my doubts and fears resurfaced. I called the urologist and then raced to the drugstore, getting there just before it closed, to pick up a prescription for Keflex, 250 mg., an antibiotic. Apparently it is just some sort of infection.

August 23, 1980

Dan has been resting quietly all day. Tonight his temperature is nearing normal. I feel so relieved.

■   ■   ■

Dan was allowed to return to work on September 2 though he was still under the surgeon's care. After his October 8 checkup and additional tests, the doctor said everything looked good. He released Dan with instructions only to return for another checkup in six months.

This was the word we had waited for! We marked our calendar to call for an appointment in March 1981 and offered a special prayer of thanksgiving at dinner.

Life once again was normal, except that never had we so appreciated each day—and each day free from pain. We resumed all of our usual activities; even so, we both felt some apprehension about Dan's first day back on the golf course, for it was here that the pain had first appeared. I waited anxiously for his return and could not hide my feelings of relief when he said he was tired and rusty, but otherwise he felt great.

With all the tests and his surgery, we had not taken any vacation during the year, so Thanksgiving week found us in Carmel, our favorite spot in all the world and the place where we had honeymooned. We spent long hours walking through the shops and galleries. Carrying our shoes, we strolled the beach, stopping now and again to take pictures, or for a brief rest. Loaded with cameras, binoculars, and food, we drove through the Carmel Valley and visited Point Lobos State Park, photographing the waves, the otters frolicking in the sheltered coves, sea lions sunning themselves on the rocks, birds scrambling for bits of lunch, and squirrels trying to quench their thirst by drinking from a dripping faucet. Then on to Big Sur and Nepenthe where we browsed the shops and sat for a time enjoying a beer while watching the waves. A red-tailed hawk which was circling the coastal mountains was too fast to catch, even in the telephoto lens, though we spent several minutes trying.

We enjoyed leisurely dinners at Neil De Vaughn's on Cannery Row where we arrived early one night to find a spectacular warehouse fire in progress. Dan ran back to the car for his camera and got some exciting shots. Like lovers, we lingered over after-dinner drinks in the Garden Room of the Highlands Inn overlooking the ocean.

On Thanksgiving Day we had so much to be thankful for! Dan was well. He had no pain. He seemed to have plenty of energy. In our holiday mood, we celebrated to the fullest. Waiting for our table at June Simpson's, we visited with the bartender, an old acquaintance from our years at the Crosby golf tournaments. We stuffed ourselves on splendid dinners of turkey with all the trimmings, accompanied by a bottle of the best Cabernet Sauvignon and concluding with mince pie and coffee. We groaned as we walked back to the hotel and tumbled into bed. Holding each other close, we slept until morning.

En route home, we stopped at Bay Meadows for a day at the races. We followed our usual practice of getting only reserved seats in the grandstand, for we liked to study the papers and the racing form, then walk down to the paddock to see the horses being saddled, hike back up to the pari-mutuel windows to make our wagers, then return to our seats to watch the race. Dan hit a daily double and we left the track with more money than when we arrived. I was amazed at his stamina. It was just like old times!

December arrived with torrents of rain, keeping us off the golf course but not interfering with the year-end festivities. We attended the lodge installation and Christmas programs, visited friends and attended a concert. The camera club held its annual awards dinner and Dan was surprised and proud to be high-point winner in his class for the year. He had entered every competition, sometimes in both slides and prints, and had won firsts for his "Moonrise" and "Blowin' It Up," second for his "Beanstream" and a third for his "One-quarter Rainbow."

I took delivery on my new IBM typewriter and Dan moved my old machine and set up an office for himself in the corner of the bedroom. He had "things he wanted to say." Obviously, no hour of his retirement, when it came, was to be wasted.

We celebrated Christmas twice with Dan's mother—first at the convalescent hospital Christmas party and again on Christmas Day. After his father's death, his mother had continued to live in Reno and we had made many weekend trips each year to visit her. In 1972 when she fell and broke her leg, Dan was on the road eleven consecutive weekends, leaving immediately after work each Friday night and returning late Sunday, a five hundred mile round trip, seeing to her care. This grueling schedule was repeated in 1974 when she fell again, but in 1978 when a stroke left her severely disabled we moved her to a convalescent hospital near us. We could no longer stand the strain of those long weekend drives ourselves.

Our own Christmas celebration started Christmas Eve and after attending church we opened our gifts. Our greatest gift, however, was the return of Dan's health. All else paled by comparison!

Phase 2: Symptoms Reappear

December 28, 1980

When we returned from church this morning, Dan complained of pain in his left hip. A knot formed in my stomach. My first thought was the cancer has come back. Was he thinking that, too? I searched his face, but he gave no evidence of any special concern.

We recapped the weekend's activities, seeking an explanation. Friday he had dethatched both the back and front lawns. I remembered that the day was warm and that he had perspired profusely. I tried to slow him down, but he was determined to complete the job.

Saturday we had gone to San Francisco to see the musical *Eubie* and to do some shopping. Walking on cement is always tiring. Was it simply overexertion? I will have to learn not to associate every pain with cancer. Dan does not express any such fear, yet he did say that he wondered if he should have continued in line at lodge to assume the office of High Priest next year. Is he doubting, too?

"Let's finish," I said firmly. "You've worked so hard and you deserve the honor."

January 5, 1981

Though six months have not yet passed, barely four, Dan had an appointment today with the urologist. The pain in his hip continues. He says it is a different type of pain, and it's in a different location. Still, it's disquieting.

He said the doctor had been noncommittal, but that he had blood tests and is to have x-rays tomorrow. Perhaps we will learn more then.

Another sleepless night.

January 6, 1981

Dan's return visit to the doctor was brief. He simply instructed Dan to take aspirins before he plays golf and after he finishes to reduce the pain and the inflammation.

Inflammation. Is that all the tests revealed? What is the cause?

We're confused. Is the cancer flaring up again, or is this really arthritis?

■ ■ ■

Dan was installed as High Priest of the Royal Arch Masons. Rain kept him off the golf course, reducing his physical activity, but the pain persisted. He called the urologist who gave him another prescription for aspirin and codeine and set up another appointment. It, too, was brief. Dan was told to use the pain medication as needed.

The office started a van pool, so he put the old Dodge to rest and each morning and evening he walked to the corner, half a mile away, to pick up his ride. He worked every day and continued all his activities, taking the pain medicine regularly. He did not complain, but I could see he was hurting much of the time.

March 6, 1981

Dan took a day of vacation so that we could go to Berkeley to the races at Golden Gate Fields. I drove the Dodge down. He said it needed some freeway driving. While I drove, he continued to work on handicapping with the new Horse Race Analyzer calculator I gave him for Christmas.

We used valet parking to save steps and even paid extra to sit in the Turf Club. We laugh about getting old, but we both know that age is not the problem. The problem *may* be the cancer. Oh God, we thought this was behind us!

■ ■ ■

Since March was our anniversary month, Dan had also scheduled a few days vacation to be spent around home. We went to Old Sacramento to take pictures and record information for an article. Then, as his pain continued, only somewhat controlled by the medication, he scheduled a complete physical examination by his family physician, who gave him a new medication to try, Butazolidin.

[It has only been in recent months that I discovered the brief notes that Dan made during this period. As I continue the diary, I will include the thoughts and feelings that he jotted down on the appropriate days in his exact words. They give insight into his inner thoughts, fears, and triumphs.]

March 24, 1981

Dan wrote, "1 pill 3 times a day for 3 days. Missed single pill at noontime. Took at 5 and 9 P.M. On my feet a great deal. Soreness noted in inside thigh area."

March 27, 1981

"On my feet a lot today. Developed pain in thigh and behind kneecap."

March 29, 1981

"Trip to Lafayette. Walked in Briones Park. Pictures. Monday morning no pain. Good night's sleep Sunday."

Today was the quarterly get-together with our Bay Area friends. After brunch in Lafayette, everyone went to Briones Park for a day of kite flying. Dan took his camera and spent his time photographing mushrooms and trying other close-ups. We then joined the rest of the group for a walk, but they continued farther than we could go, so we returned to the car, thinking they would be along soon. The cars were locked and we had not brought our own, so we were forced to remain out in the cold until their return. We waited for more than an hour and got thoroughly chilled. I was furious with such thoughtlessness, but Dan insisted that I say nothing about it. He didn't want to spoil the group's day of fun. Somehow I must keep as calm about all this as he, but it's a struggle.

Back at the house, the conversation turned to tax shelters, vacations, and other trivia which also upset me. Dan and I are fighting for life. Other matters seem so insignificant. He took it all in stride. I thought today was much too hard on him. Too much exercise. Too much exposure to the cold March winds; however, when we got home he took his pain medicine and slept well.

Am I being overprotective?

April 2, 1981

"In evening, pain in muscle of thigh going down to kneecap. Woke up in night. Took aspirin and put on heating pad and went back to sleep."

April 3, 1981
  "Still feel pain in muscle and kneecap."

April 5, 1981
  "Began new course of medicine. 1 tablet 3 times a day. Motrin."

April 11, 1981
  "3:10 A.M. Pain in groin, knee and in left ankle. Took 2 aspirins and got the heating pad. Still pain. Got up at 4:20 A.M. No relief.
  "5:50 A.M. took Motrin, milk and breakfast. Relief began at 6:30 A.M. Played golf. Motrin with lunch. After, bath and soak. Afternoon nap. Motrin with dinner."

April 12, 1981
  "6:40 A.M. Up. No pain. Only stiffness from exercise."

April 16, 1981
  "Still feeling great! Free from pain."
  Tonight we attended the Maundy Thursday Communion Service and as we listened to the music and meditated while waiting for our turn to visit the Upper Room, I shared my concern with God. *Please don't let the cancer return. Please make Dan well again.* I'm so grateful for the periods of ease and the freedom from pain but so fearful of its recurrence and the way it seems to spread from place to place. Yet Dan seems confident with this new medication. I must pledge my faith with his. We both had tears in our eyes as we partook of the bread and the wine, the symbols of Christ's suffering for us; but Sunday brings Easter, spring, and we can look forward to a new beginning.

■ ■ ■

  For the next six weeks the Motrin, an anti-inflammatory drug used for treatment of arthritis, kept Dan relatively free from pain. During that time we spent a week's vacation in Southern California where he attended the state meeting of Royal Arch Masons and was initiated into the Order of the High Priesthood. He attended long days of meetings and we enjoyed the dinner dances and evening entertainment. Before returning home, we spent a day at the J. Paul Getty Museum in Malibu and a day at the races at Hollywood Park. En route home we stayed over in Santa Barbara, went sightseeing and photographing at Solvang and the missions of Santa Inez and Lompoc. It was a busy time and I noticed his heavy sweating at night, but otherwise he seemed fine. We were encouraged.

Back at home he was at work every day and each Monday he joined two of his buddies to play in the company-sponsored golf league. This trio had brought many a trophy home. After much exertion, Dan did experience pain from time to time, but the Motrin always made it go away, so our spirits continued to be uplifted. We lived a day at a time and filled each moment with work and play, meetings and projects, always looking toward the future when Dan could retire and we would both work seriously at photography and writing.

We slept like a teaspoon inside a tablespoon as we had since our marriage began; we cuddled and were never closer. The lack of fulfillment was frustrating but neither of us let on. Dan was just thankful to be alive and I vowed to do nothing to destroy his confidence or self-esteem.

May 23, 1981

Dan gave up his usual golf today to participate in the camera club field trip. The weather was warm and the sweat just poured from him. He was tired and sore after the day's outing and the Motrin gave him no relief. His leg hurts so bad. He will call his regular physician Monday.

What next? I'm so worried. The word *metastases* did appear on the surgery papers. That means the cancer had spread before it gave any symptoms or was detected. How extensive is it? Has the cessation of testosterone production failed to stop it? Is the cancer traveling now?

May 28, 1981

The doctor's charge slip shows a diagnosis of "calf muscle pull"; however, Dan is to have lab work done and return next week.

June 2, 1981

Today's charge slip also shows "calf muscle pull," but more lab work was done. Dan said the doctor told him to take things a little easier and to continue with the medication.

"Is that all?"

"Yes," Dan shrugged. "Perhaps he doesn't know either. I'll slow down a bit and see if that helps."

Again I tell myself not to associate every ache and pain with cancer, but what else can it be? And why doesn't the doctor say?

June 26, 1981

Dorothy and I left early this morning for Mills College in Oakland to attend the California Writers' Club seminar. Upon arriving, I discovered she had put Dan's briefcase into the trunk, thinking it was mine. It contained all the papers and instructions for his meeting tonight and one tomorrow in Comptche. He was to preside over both functions. When the error was discovered, she offered to drive all the way back, but I phoned Dan. As usual, he kept his cool, told me to open the case and give him some information he had written down. He asked questions. I located the answers among his files and he made notes. He assured us he could get along without the briefcase. I was almost in tears at his patience and understanding. Dorothy was moved, too, and sensed something more was wrong. I decided to share with her the fears that Dan and I are facing. Outside of the immediately family, we have confided in only three couples of close friends. There is such a stigma attached to cancer and the doctors have not yet acknowledged that cancer is our current problem. Whatever it is, we can fight it. We can win. The fact that the pain will not stay away, however, is becoming a constant nagging worry.

July 17, 1981

I met Dan at the Bloomington, Illinois airport at 9 A.M. His face was grey with fatigue and pain as he got off the tiny hedge-hopper that runs between Chicago and downstate Illinois, following his night flight from San Francisco. He looked so haggard and miserable, my heart very nearly stopped. I drove back to Mom's, he took his medicine, had a nap and seemed to be fully recovered.

■　■　■

The next days were spent in the bosom of my family. Dan's color was not always good and he was frequently drenched with perspiration, but then the weather was hot and humid. He was in good humor and did not complain. We took day trips throughout Lincoln land, taking pictures and gathering information for articles, and when it was time to leave, we took a compartment on the train to see the country once more.

It was the first overland trip either of us had made in many years. We both enjoyed experiencing once again the immensity of the land, the diverse geography. Like a couple of kids, we got off the train in Denver and bought ice cream cones in the station. In Wyoming, we saw a herd of elk right near the tracks. We roamed hand-in-hand near the station in Rawlins and reminisced about the two miserable weeks we had spent there at the time of our accident, back in 1954.

I tried to visualize how the land had looked when my great-great-grandmother Isabel, whose biography I was writing, made this same journey in 1871. Dan assisted in the creation of the illusion with his knowledge of history and geography.

When he did not feel well, he simply took some medicine and lay down. We savored each moment and tried not to think of what might lie ahead.

August 14, 1981

This was Dan's final day of vacation. He had made arrangements to join his Hackers and Slicers Golf group for their annual outing to Aptos Seascape Golf Course. We had reservations at the Holiday Inn in Santa Cruz so drove down Thursday evening after work.

While Dan played golf, I went sightseeing and sketching in Capitola. After the festivities were over and the prizes awarded, we started home, stopping to visit some friends in San Jose and ended up staying for dinner. We left immediately after the meal and I could see that Dan was agitated. As soon as we were out of the congestion of city traffic, he asked me to drive. This was most unusual. The remainder of the trip home was a nightmare. I have never seen anyone in so much agony. He was in such excruciating pain that he climbed all over the car—back seat, front seat, kneeling, almost standing, crouching, as he tried to get comfortable and could not. I drove as fast as I dared, but it seemed an eternity before we got home.

He took his pain medicine, plugged in the heating pad and went to bed. Eventually he got a little rest.

Something has to be done. He cannot continue in such pain! The Motrin and the aspirin and codeine together do not help. Surely arthritis would not be this painful. The cancer must have returned.

August 18, 1981

Dan saw his urologist today. He now has the results of the bone scan which was done August 4—an imaging of Dan's entire body. At the time it sounded ominous, but we put our fears on hold and waited for the results and for the blood work. Now we know. The cancer is again active. I suspect it has been all along, but the doctors didn't say. Dan has been advised to contact a radiologist for possible radiation treatments. He has an appointment in two days.

I wonder at his calm. I know nothing about radiation but the cancer is frightening enough. Still, we must keep positive for life to be bearable. *Dear God, may I find the strength and the courage to support Dan through this anxious time.*

August 20, 1981

After work, Dan paid his first visit to the radiologist for consultation and examination. He brought home a pamphlet which explains radiation therapy.

"A new chapter in the dramatic story of how radiation therapy is saving lives of cancer patients is about to be written."

This opening paragraph was most encouraging!

Dan, in his usual thorough manner, questioned the radiologist at length. What about exercise? Golf? Hiking? Walking? Use of alcohol? Any special diet? Do's and don'ts while under treatment? Schedule of treatments?

All of his questions were answered to his satisfaction. Apparently, he can continue living a "normal" life. He does not even seem concerned about the possible side effects, which he said were upset stomach, loss of hair, and skin irritation. He likes this young doctor and is convinced these new treatments will take care of his problem.

Another blood panel is to be done and the series of treatments is to begin August 31.

I cannot help but share Dan's enthusiasm. I know that major strides have been made in cancer treatment. Since the surgery itself was not enough, surely the radiation will complete his cure.

Phase 3: Radiation, New Therapy for Dan

September 22, 1981

At 9 A.M., Dan had his first radiation treatment on his left hip, then went on to work. I tried to keep busy, but my thoughts were on him all day. *I'm frightened of the disease and of the treatment.* Radiation destroys. The purpose is to destroy the cancer cells, but though it is skillfully controlled, surely there is opportunity for damage to surrounding tissue.

When he came home, he was enthusiastic. He showed me the area which had been outlined to guide the technician. He had experienced no discomfort except that of lying still on the hard table, but it was only for a brief time. Subsequent treatments will be given late in the afternoon so that he will not have to take any more time off from work. A series of twenty treatments has been scheduled, four times a week for five weeks. Wednesday is to be his day off. Two new medications have been added by the radiologist: Talwin for pain and Donnatal in the event Dan should suffer an upset stomach.

God, please let the radiation stop the cancer's spread and put an end to Dan's pain.

■ ■ ■

Dan's radiation therapy was delayed for three weeks. It was a time of anxiety, frustration and additional confusion as we faced still a different crisis. When he came home from work on Friday, August 21, his face was flushed and he had a fever. All weekend his temperature was over 100°, sometimes as high as 103°. His abdominal area was tender and he had been constipated for several days. He saw his family physician who prescribed 250 mg. of tetracycline for this spell of "diverticulitus." Dulcolax, Milk of Magnesia and Metamucil were also recommended.

The fever persisted and he lost five pounds in two days. 500 mg. of tetracycline was tried. The fever continued. In addition to feeling miserable, Dan was severely disappointed to have plans for the radiation treatments postponed. They would not begin until the fever was under control. We were on hold.

I was concerned about the possible side effects of all the different medications. I wrote for Public Affairs pamphlets, *Know Your Medication* and *Drugs—Use, Misuse, Abuse Guidance for Families.*

The fever was accompanied by drenching sweats which stained the bedclothes and his pajamas yellow. The diagnosis still read "diverticulitis," but Dan had additional blood tests. Amoxicillyn, 500 mg., was prescribed.

Now nausea was added to his other symptoms. I wondered if the upset stomach was a result of the massive doses of medication he had been taking over such a long period of time. He was still taking 1,800 mg. of Motrin daily, in addition to the new antibiotics and some pain medicine. The urinalysis and barium enema with x-rays made of his abdomen proved negative. The diagnosis was now "Fever of an Unknown Cause."

Dan had talked with his former doctor in Berkeley. He was involved with three doctors here, his family physician, the urologist and the radiologist. It gave him a sense of comfort to talk over his problems with the one doctor who had known him over a period of years. The fever, still unexplained, continued for several more days.

At the end of the first week of radiation treatments, our spirits were high. Dan's pain was quieting down and thus far he had experienced none of the possible reactions.

In the meantime, it was our turn to entertain our Bay Area friends. Dan insisted he felt up to the occasion. We made plans for a picnic at Fieldstone Winery and as he noted on his calendar, "Great Time!"

The radiologist had said to "live normally but with care." No stress or strain. We readily understood that the radiation was killing cells, both healthy and diseased, and that weakness would result. I was at all times concerned about Dan hurting himself, lifting anything heavy, twisting getting into and out of the car. Logic told us that the left hip area which was getting treatment would be extremely vulnerable. He was still taking the Motrin daily, bolstered by Talwin as needed for pain, but the pain was being controlled and that gave us encouragement. We were confident that the radiation would stop the cancer in the area to which it had spread and that there would be no additional problems.

In addition to the information given to us by the radiologist, we picked up a copy of the pamphlet *Radiation Therapy and You*, published by the U.S. Department of Health and Human Services. Dan was undergoing external radiation therapy in which the machine, at some distance from his body, beamed the high energy rays to the cancer. Radiation destroys the ability of all cells within its reach, cancerous and normal, to grow and reproduce. Cancer cells, however, are more susceptible to its effect. Usual reaction to treatment is fatigue, loss of appetite and skin irritation, nausea or diarrhea, loss of hair. The effects vary from patient to patient depending somewhat upon the area being treated. So far Dan had had no reactions.

October 6, 1981
      Dan wrote, "7:45 A.M. Knees stiff. General aches. Stiff knees and achy. Moving gingerly. Shooting pains like darts from groin to left hip. Evening after treatment, developed pain in both sides of pelvis. Took Talwin at 7:15 P.M. and another at 7:45. No effect. Up three times within forty-five minutes, then slept fine until 2 A.M. Woke up from drenching sweat. Back to sleep until 4 A.M."

October 7, 1981
      "Woke up with no pain in pelvic area. Still stiff in knees but feel much better. Did I walk too much at work on Monday? Felt better all afternoon. Pain and stiffness left. Didn't walk as much at work today. No pain pills. Hurrah! This may just be the start of a better life."

October 8, 1981
      "Still move gingerly. Soreness in buttocks is dull. Left pelvic area began pain and throb early afternoon. Took two Talwin at 7 P.M. Worked good but made me woozy. Bed by 8:30 P.M. Awake at 10. Took another Talwin. 1 A.M. awoke with severe pain in right thigh muscle. Believe I've caught cold or else virus has attacked that muscle. Took codeine and aspirin and slept until 6 A.M."

October 14, 1981

"Fine start. No medicine other than Motrin. Catch in right thigh not as noticeable. At noon throbbing in right thigh muscle resumed. Painful and feels like I'd fall down. Also have pain in lower right back. Temperature jumped to 101° at 7:30 P.M. but was normal within an hour."

October 16, 1981

Today after work, Dan had the fourteenth of twenty radiation treatments on his left hip, but as a result of yesterday's x-rays, plans have been made to begin treating the right hip next week, a total of fourteen treatments. Another setback! The radiologist described it as another hot area. But Dan insists the treatments are helping his left side. He seems confident they will also help the right. Fear keeps nagging at me.

Dear God, do not let Dan sense my fears. Please help me to find the same faith and courage that sustains him.

■   ■   ■

For the next two weeks, Dan received two radiation treatments each visit, one on each hip until the first series was completed October 29. The series on the right hip was completed November 12.

While we celebrated the end of the radiation treatments, all was not well. The pain continued. We were hopeful, but we were concerned. Dan went to work every day. He had lost weight, but he looked fit. He continued participating in lodge and in camera club but he did not attempt golf. Though weekends were now only for church and rest, we did continue some social life. At a fund-raiser for a local arts center, Dan saw two of his golfing partners. He assured them he would be back on the fairways soon.

We received our order blank for tickets to the Bing Crosby Pro-Am Golf Tournament and we made plans to attend. We loved Carmel and would enjoy a visit to the area even if our time out on the courses had to be limited. We bought tickets entitling us to reserved grandstand seats at the 18th hole and made motel reservations. Living confidently was our motto.

November 18, 1981

Unsure of what we were facing, Dan prepared the following list
of questions for his appointment with the urologist:

1. What can I do to quiet my prostate? Sharp darts again into
    left side. 22 radiation treatments [actually there had been
    34] all for naught?
2. Drenching sweats are worse since radiation ceased. Does
    this show I need hormone treatments, or some such supple-
    mentary treatment program?
3. Describe how I felt after walking on cement downtown
    Saturday. Walked from Macy's garage to Consumers Dis-
    tributors on 4th, 3 blocks and back. Knees throbbed. Groin
    muscle acted like it had done from February to August
    when radiation was suggested.
4. What can I expect? Radiologist could only say be alert for
    pain.
5. I'm taking 600 units of Motrin 3 x daily. Can it hide symp-
    toms of my prostate acting up?
6. Radiologist indicated he only treated the hottest portions.
    Where else is this cancer? What can I do about it? PMA.
    [Positive Mental Attitude.] Keep up strength. Don't over-
    exert, etc.
7. What vitamins and mineral supplements should I be taking
    to put back what has been taken out from radiation treat-
    ments, Motrin, antibiotics, etc?
8. Pain medicine. When I want fast relief I use ASA with co-
    deine. When I want longer relief but I don't need it as soon,
    I use Talwin. Not constipated now and keeping regular with
    Metamucil, so I'm able to use both pain pills.

His visit with the urologist was brief. He was sent for a testosterone check, the results of which were reported later by phone. "As
expected." What does that mean? If the cessation of production of
the male hormone was to stop the cancer, why does it continue to
flare up?

Dan does not voice any concern, so I do not ask. I am frightened, but I take my cue from him and keep my fears to myself.

November 19, 1981

Today x-rays were taken of his lumbosacral spine and thoracic spine after another consultation with the radiologist. Plans were made for a new series of radiation treatments to the lower back to commence November 30, after Thanksgiving.

More disappointment, but not despair. We pray and tenaciously hold fast to the thought that this *must* be the last.

Dan brought home new information from the Radiation-Oncology Clinic for patients receiving radiation therapy to the abdominal area. It warned of possible diarrhea . Dan joked that it would be a welcome change from the constipation.

But I can't help thinking, *a third series of radiation. How much can the human body withstand?* Dan acts as if it is only a temporary setback. He seems to have such faith. I must keep my thoughts positive, too.

■ ■ ■

During the following weeks of treatment, we tried to maintain our normal routines. We went to church and gave thanks for each day and prayed for the future. We enjoyed Thanksgiving dinner at a favorite restaurant. We drove through the wine country and visited the Hollyberry Fair at Souverain and partook of the festivities at Fieldstone Winery.

December 7, 1981

Over the weekend Dan again developed a high fever so he stayed home from work this morning. I cancelled my writers' workshop and accompanied him for his fifth radiation treatment on his lower back. It was my first visit to the Radiation-Oncology Clinic. I found it frightening. The attendants were kind and considerate, but the massive equipment and the warning signs posted everywhere gave me a chill. This entire subject of radiation, even in therapy, is awesome to me. Can it really be adequately controlled? Does it work? But I share Dan's enthusiasm for the radiologist. He is warm, understanding and easy to talk with. I told him I thought he needed two more specialists in his clinic, a nutrition expert and a physical therapist. It seems to me that some special diet or dietary supplement combined with a supervised exercise program is necessary to help the body to rebuild and restore itself.

The doctor sent Dan for a blood test and platelet count. He is now anemic. Ferancee-HP pills, an iron and vitamin C supplement, have been added to his list of medications.

He will, however, return to work tomorrow.

December 17, 1981

"4:30 A.M. Woke with a pain in my chest as if my ribs were being squeezed. My eyes, face and left hand are swollen. Am I allergic to something? Things I've been taking all along—Motrin, Metamucil, prunes, Talwin, aspirin and codeine. Things I've added—iron pills, high-potency multi vitamins with minerals."

Later Dan could not get his breath and we made a hurried dash to the emergency room at the hospital. The doctor there gave him shots of Benadryl and adrenalin and did an electrocardiogram, which was normal. After his radiation treatment, we stopped to see his family physician who gave him another shot of adrenalin and a prescription for oral Benadryl.

Though Dan felt somewhat better, he could not keep down his supper. He took the Benadryl and went to bed at 6:30. He seems so weak tonight, yet only yesterday he looked great and we were feeling really positive. These ups and downs are frustrating. Dan laughs that he is like Job and his boils. I try to keep it light, but my heart is heavy.

■ ■ ■

The radiation treatments, the allergic reactions and the additional medication used to control them so weakened Dan that he was unable to return to work. Each morning he tried, but his fever continued and before he finished breakfast, he would realize that he was not yet strong enough.

I tried to find the cause of his allergies. I checked the warning sheets for each prescription. What Dan was experiencing was described as a possible reaction to Motrin, though a rare one; but the first reaction appeared to have been triggered by the iron pills. He had also recently reacted to Talwin. The iron pills contained yellow dye. So did the multivitamins he had taken. I called our druggist. Was there yellow dye in Motrin and Talwin? The answer was yes. I thought I had discovered the cause of the allergies.

I had read in the paper about the possible introduction of legislation to permit the use of heroin to treat patients with extreme problems of pain, such as cancer patients experience, and Dan helped me to compose a letter to our senators asking their support of such legislation. We felt there were so many allergic reactions and side effects from medications that the doctor and the patient should be free to select and use whatever was the most effective.

We celebrated Christmas with Dan's mother at the convalescent hospital and I took pictures of the two of them together. Dan was smiling with his arm around his mother and he looked so healthy. It was sometimes difficult to realize all he was going through. At home we had a quiet day. I fixed duck with a cranberry glaze, one of Dan's favorite meals, and for dessert we had pumpkin pie with Cool Whip. Next morning he had another allergic reaction. I checked the list of ingredients on the Cool Whip container. Sure enough, it contained yellow dye. We then ordered a Medic-Alert bracelet stating Dan's allergies to yellow dyes #5 and 6, as we both believed they were the culprits.

And so the year ended. The medication controlled the allergic reactions when they occurred, but they seemed to be lessened when all yellow dye was eliminated. The best news was that the radiation treatments would soon be coming to an end. When they were finished, Dan would regain his strength and his health.

We held our own New Year's Eve service at home, each adding a prayer to our usual daily devotions with the *Upper Room* and the *Daily Word* and retired early.

Dan's last radiation treatment on his lower back was January 5 and he hoped to return to work shortly thereafter. He had even made an appointment to check in with the company doctor on January 6 with his release; but when he discussed his condition with the radiologist, they both felt he was as yet too weak to work. Dan needed some time without treatment to give his body opportunity to rebuild.

January 8, 1982

"2 P.M., opened chapter. 9 P.M., bed with 2 Tylenol and codeine."

Dan's brief notes do not tell the drama of this day, for today brought another disappointment. Tonight was the installation of officers for his Royal Arch Masonic Lodge. In spite of fighting his disease, he has attended all the meetings this year and as outgoing High Priest, he has desperately hoped he would be able to preside at this, his last meeting, in that capacity. He had written his speech and I had typed it for him. He had also written a proxy letter in the event he was unable to attend.

At 2 P.M., I drove him to the lodge hall and he, with the other officers, went through the formalities of Opening Chapter. When we returned home from those few minutes, less than an hour in all, it was obvious he was not strong enough to attend the evening function. His face was pale and he was soaked with perspiration. I tried to conceal my heartbreak and temporarily hold back the tears. I called the lodge brother who was to be his proxy. He came over to pick up Dan's speech and his letter of apology at not being able to appear in person. We were all three in tears by the time he left the house.

■ ■ ■

The days became all alike with Dan at home. He was up for breakfast and to read the paper, then returned to bed for a nap; up for lunch, followed by an afternoon nap, dinner and early to bed. The pain medicines kept him drowsy and we both knew the rest would do him good. He needed plenty of food and sleep to rebuild his body which had been subjected to such extensive abuse by the radiation and the cancer. Saturday and Sunday were no different from any other days, except that I continued to go to church. While I worshipped in the sanctuary, he worshipped at home, bolstering our faith, our strength and our courage. During the week I would slip out for a few hours to visit his mother in the convalescent hospital. The pain and the sweating that awakened Dan frequently during the night interfered with our rest. By the time I changed the bed each time, it was difficult to return to sleep.

He picked up our cat, a hefty twelve-pounder, and strained his back. The radiologist prescribed liquid morphine for this new pain and suggested x-rays. Vertebrae T 3–9 were "hot." Another series of radiation began. How many more could he take? To learn that the cancer had once more spread increased my anxiety. I silently wondered if it would ever stop. Dan did not record any such feeling. He simply accepted and coped. He acted as if it would stop! It had to stop!

I wrote to the motel in Carmel and cancelled our reservations for the Crosby.

January 20, 1982

Dan awoke with nausea again this morning and he discontinued all vitamins. At his third radiation treatment, the radiologist gave him a prescription for Compazine for the nausea. He told Dan to continue with the liquid morphine and methadone pills for pain. He had trouble keeping his medicine down during the day but tonight he was able to retain three methadone pills and got some sleep.

Today is my birthday. In-between doctors' appointments, I went to the hairdresser. Friends came by for a birthday drink. Dan, who has not been out of the house except to go to the clinic or to the doctor's office since Christmas Day, delivered this hand-printed card this morning at breakfast:

PRIEST'S BANK   01-04/536   #1
Dover Ct. Branch   1210 (1)
Santa Rosa, CA 95401
                                   Jan. 20, 1982
Pay to the order of MARY PRIEST
RAIN CHECK to be redeemed for 1 gift, 1 dinner,
or 1 other type of entertainment selected by Payee.
                                   Daniel H. Priest

We clung to each other when he gave it to me and I tried to hide my tears. I'm sure I shall never receive a birthday card that I treasure as much as this.

January 26, 1982

"Up at 6. Vitamin B-12 shot at 2 P.M. Radiation at 2:40 P.M. Visited Mom. Didn't recognize me. Dinner 6 P.M. Bed 10. Still no strong painkiller other than Tylenol."

Dan's terse notes do not convey what must have been the depth of his emotions at his experience. He was feeling better and so, following his radiation treatment, he suggested we stop by the con-valescent hospital to visit his mother. He had not seen her since Christmas.

She was seated in her wheelchair near the front window when we arrived and she acknowledged me as usual. I put an arm around her and said, "Look, Ellen, Dan's come to see you."

She looked up at him and shook her head, no. She whimpered and fussed as he tried to talk with her and hold her hand. She pulled away from him and insisted that she didn't know him. A nurse came by and said it was because of Ellen's condition; that she could have forgotten Dan in the month's interval. I cannot accept that explanation. Dan's appearance has changed little during that time in spite of the hell he has been through. We both know of Ellen's cancer phobia. Whenever she gets any ailment, she is sure it's cancer and becomes almost hysterical until a visit to her doctor can allay her fears. I'm convinced that this fear is what caused her to act as if she didn't recognize her own son.

What it did to Dan, making the supreme effort in his weakened condition, and facing this life-threatening illness himself, to visit his mother and then to be totally rejected by her, I can only imagine. He seemed, however, to shrug it off.

I was encouraged that he had felt well enough to go to visit her. These past few days, he has seemed stronger and occasionally takes his camera outside and takes pictures. Sometimes he stays up with me, watching television. Just looking over at him relaxing in his big chair gives me a sense of peace.

January 27, 1982

"Day off from radiation. Took some pictures. Felt much better. Dinner 6:30 P.M. Bed 11:00 P.M."

January 28, 1982

"Up at 6:15 A.M. Took Donnatal at 7:15 and Tylenol at 7:30. Noon, lost feeling in left leg and motor control of left arm and hand. 2:40 P.M., radiation, saw Dr. David. Told him these symptoms usually clear up in 5 or 6 hours. 5 P.M. cocktails—gin martini. 7:30 dinner; 10:30 bed with 2 Tylenol. Up at 1:30 and took 2 aspirin. Couldn't sleep. Stayed up until 3:45. Bed again 3:45 A.M. Leg and arm still not recovered."

Phase 4: Acute Care Hospital Stay

January 29, 1982
"Up 7:45 A.M. 1 aspirin. 8:30 breakfast."

■ ■ ■

Before the morning was over, our world collapsed around our shoulders. He arose from his stool at the breakfast counter, took a faltering step and slid to the floor. I tried to help him up but he pushed me away. I asked if I could get one of the neighbors to give him a hand.

"No!" He was adamant. "Call an ambulance."

I have become so ingrained with the need to keep calm, not to panic when things go wrong, that even with his request, I hesitated. I wondered who to call. He hadn't seen his family physician for several weeks. Since we have better communications with the radiologist, and we saw him only yesterday, I decided to call the radiology clinic. They advised me to call his family physician and an ambulance.

The ambulance service responded immediately, sirens screaming an alarm which added to our fright. The attendants checked Dan briefly, loaded him on a stretcher and started to the hospital. I followed in our car.

By the time we reached the hospital, Dan was in a full seizure similar to that of an epileptic, head rolling, eyes unable to focus, mouth open, and all the time his body jerked uncontrollably. These jerking movements caused him excruciating pain. I was frantic! I could imagine the agony he was suffering. The aides in the emergency room acted as if Dan were in the throes of a simple epileptic seizure and when I tried to explain his condition to them, they dismissed me and insisted that I wait outside. I took care of the paperwork at the desk and then forced my way back into the examining room.

It seemed an eternity before anything was done to help him. Where was his doctor? He needed someone who knew his physical problems. I was the only one in the room who knew Dan's condition and obviously no one would pay attention to me.

Intravenous injections of Valium were started when the doctor arrived. The seizures continued, affecting Dan's entire left side. More Valium. Finally the movements lessened as the medicine took effect, and he was more comfortable. Dan was to be admitted to the hospital for diagnosis and treatment, but as there were no beds immediately available, we spent the morning in the emergency room. Shortly after 1 P.M., he was taken into a two-bed room.

From there the nightmare continued as he was whisked in and out of bed, in and out of his room, hauled about like a sack of grain, for various tests. A CAT-scan, electroencephalogram, x-rays. I was not informed as to what was going on and I paced up and down the halls, waiting, waiting, waiting to be acknowledged and included. For almost twenty-nine years we have been together, faced every challenge and problem and heartache together. I was frustrated and furious at being excluded from this, our most serious trauma thus far. I knew only that Dan was in desperate pain, that he had experienced something like a stroke. Why? What had caused it? What could be done about it?

I didn't even know when his physician left to go back to his office.

When Dan was returned from X-ray, a catheter had been inserted. The nurse told me he had trouble urinating and the catheter was used to save time so that they could proceed immediately with the tests.

My heart ached as I watched him lie in bed, the pain caused by the involuntary movements of those disease-ridden bones etched in his face. His mouth now had a slight droop in the left corner. His left hand was clenched into a fist which he could not release. His left foot was turned under in an unnatural position. He had very little control of or feeling in the entire left side of his body. Dilantin, phenobarbital and Decadron, the usual medications for seizures, were now being administered.

By evening he was more quiet and comfortable, but we still did not know what we were now facing. Our radiologist came by the hospital and I told him of my worries and concerns. He called a neurologist for us and I overheard part of his conversation. "Keep the family informed," he instructed this new specialist.

An unexpected blessing in this unspeakable day was the arrival of Dan's brother Charles, here on a business trip to the Bay Area. We hadn't expected to see him this trip, but he had finished his work early, so he rented a car and drove up. Arriving at our house and finding no one at home, he learned from a neighbor where to find us. Now, at least we are not alone. We have some family support.

The neurologist arrived, examined Dan and looked at the tests already done. He saw nothing conclusive. He ordered another CAT-scan and allowed Charles and me to accompany Dan in the ambulance to the clinic to be with him during the test. Dan was injected with more Valium to keep him sedated during the procedure. By comparing the earlier test with this one, the neurologist spotted the problem: a "hot spot" that was putting pressure on Dan's brain, causing the seizures. The cancer has once again metastasized. As soon as the seizures are controlled, this new area can be treated with radiation.

We returned to the hospital. A friend from Dan's office stopped by and Dan made the introductions. "This is my brother, the double-dipper," he said, alluding to Charles's retired status from the Navy and his present work for a firm that did business with the Navy.

Charles convinced me to go home to bed. He would stay the night with Dan.

I did, but I cannot sleep. I marvel at Dan's sense of humor and his optimism. He was relieved to know he had not suffered a stroke and he is anxious to get the new treatments started. His confidence is contagious and I try to share his optimism, but I remember that a few times in recent weeks, he has mentioned a lack of feeling in his left leg, or his arm or hand, "like it had gone to sleep." I have also noticed occasional mental lapses when he would be sitting in his chair, almost asleep, and talk of someone or some occasion from the past that I knew nothing about. I have attributed such occurrences to the effects of the strong pain medicine. *Dear God, please don't let that bright, incisive mind be impaired by this latest episode! I don't think I could stand it.*

■ ■ ■

Dan's brother left to return to his home in Virginia. I stayed with Dan both day and night. The neurologist said he should not be left alone as he was so highly medicated, partially paralyzed and with little coordination. He was unable to call the nurse and his room was some distance from the nurses' station. Then the neighbors set up shifts to stay with Dan during the night, allowing me to get some rest, until he could be left alone.

February 4, 1982

The new series of radiation treatments to Dan's skull was started today. The ambuvan came by the hospital about 9:30 A.M. Dan was lifted from the bed to the wheelchair, still with the catheter. Wrapped in blankets, he, in his wheelchair, was locked into place in the van, while I rode up front with the driver. It is only a block from the hospital to the radiology clinic. The driver stayed with us, waiting during the brief treatment, then returned us to the hospital. The treatments are to be four days each week. Now, we were warned that with radiation to the skull, Dan will surely lose that thick, black hair.

■ ■ ■

Our days settled into a routine. I went to the hospital each day by 8 A.M. to help Dan with his breakfast and to prepare his menu for the following day. Then we went to the clinic for radiation. We had lunch together, usually a brown bag for me, though sometimes I ordered a guest tray from the hospital kitchen. In the afternoons we both dozed. When he was awake, we talked quietly of the future. This was one more setback we would have to overcome. Together, and with God's help, we could win this battle, too. I left only after he was asleep each night.

During these long days and nights in the hospital, we yearned for the old days of private rooms. Not solely because of the lack of privacy, but more importantly because Dan's roommates were so disturbing. His first roommate was a young man who had had back surgery and was soon to be discharged. He was mobile and pleasant, but he had many visitors who smoked incessantly. The next was an elderly man, somewhat senile, who was suffering from cancer of the bladder. He, too, was mobile; in fact, the nurses had great difficulty finding him and keeping him in bed. He was up and down, in and out, running around the halls.

But the last roommate was the most depressing, an older man who had attempted suicide by shotgun and left himself a vegetable. Whenever I was with Dan, I would draw the curtains between the two beds. Every time the nurses came in, they opened them. The sight was almost more than I could bear. Worse was the irony. Dan was fighting, struggling, exerting every fiber of his being to live, and he was trapped in a room with what was left of this gentleman who had so desperately wanted to die that he had tried to take his own life.

Meanwhile, plants and flowers poured in from neighbors and friends from work and lodge. Dan had many visitors. His department at work sent him a huge poster with floral designs and messages signed by everyone. We put it up on the wall, and the doctors and nurses added their signatures. The daily visits of our pastor brought enormous comfort.

Most of all, Dan cherished the card and letter he received from my mother:

> Just a word to tell you I am praying for your speedy recovery. I'm so sorry that I can't be there or be of any help to you or Mary. I hope you are more comfortable today, but don't forget it takes time, and sometimes it does seem endless, I know. I think of you as a son and love you just as much.
>
> Ara

X-rays were taken of both of Dan's legs to determine how soon he could start physical therapy. The neurologist showed me how to stretch Dan's left foot to try to work it back into a normal position. We were encouraged that some movement was returning to his left arm. He constantly massaged his clenched left fist. Radiation treatments were resumed on his upper back so that each visit to the clinic resulted in a double dose of radiation. Another electroencephalogram was done to check his progress.

When physical therapy started, I accompanied Dan to each session so that I would know how to help him when he got home. No one knew if he would fully regain use of his left side. He worked so hard and endured much pain in his efforts to get back on his feet. For more than two weeks, he had required the help of two aides to lift him from bed to wheelchair. Now his days were exhausting, with radiation treatments each morning and physical therapy each afternoon. He worked with silly putty to strengthen his hands and endlessly squeezed a rubber ball. His face was tense with the pain all the exertion caused him, but he was determined.

Meanwhile, life went on in the outside world. Dan was responsible for his mother's business affairs. He had her power of attorney, he was a signator on her bank and savings accounts and he could take care of her business so long as he was able to act. Now her bills had to be paid. I brought her checkbook to the hospital and helped Dan to sign several blank checks so I could take care of these.

But taking care of her business led us to think of our own. We talked about our wills, and when I looked them over I found they were woefully out of date. I took them to the hospital and Dan and I discussed the changes needed. I called and set up an appointment with our attorney. I felt physically ill as I kept the appointment. It was as if in these preparations I was exhibiting a lack of faith in Dan's recovery, a lack of confidence that we would really see this through. It was almost as if I were casting an evil spell over us. Why did we wait until a crisis arose?

February 18, 1982

When I walked into Dan's room this morning, he said, "The doctor wants you to call him."

I thought it might be about Dan's going home, though we had received no previous warning. I talked with his nurses and therapists. All of them said, "Mrs. Priest, there is no way you can take care of him by yourself."

I returned to Dan's room and we discussed his homecoming. We both wanted him to stay in the hospital until the radiation treatments were over. He was too weak and in too much pain to withstand the long trips from our home to the clinic. He still had the catheter. They had not even tried to discontinue its use. He was up only a short time each day and he was assisted in all of his activities by two nurses or aides.

I knew we would need guard railings installed by our steps and grab bars put in the bathroom. I had already contacted a carpenter to do these things for us. I needed to contact the Department of Motor Vehicles to get a Disabled Parking Permit for future doctors' appointments. All this takes time.

When I called the doctor and explained our position, he argued a bit about hospital usage, study committees and was not overly receptive to my plea, but he, too, did not want to transfer Dan to a convalescent hospital for such a short interim. He consented to a discharge on February 25 which coincided with the last radiation treatment. He also referred me to the discharge planner for assistance.

I went to her office. She was on the phone when I entered and I waited. She said "Hello" and the phone rang again. This continued for nearly an hour. I was accomplishing nothing. Finally, with her free hand, she scooped up a collection of brochures, stuffed them into an envelope and said, "Here, study these."

When I got home from the hospital tonight, I started through the envelope. There are advertisements of various businesses who supply household help, companions, home health aides, registered nurses, and licensed vocational nurses. I don't know what we need. The nurses and therapists tell me that Dan doesn't sleep well, that he suffers from nightmares and hallucinations. He still has the catheter. He is in bed all the time, except for the trips to the radiologist, or when he takes a few steps with his walker a couple of times a day. It takes two people to help him in and out of bed. He sure isn't mobile. How can I handle him—with my weak back? My blood pressure has shot up, even though my doctor gave me a prescription for Valium, which does help me sleep.

What a challenge!

I'm scared stiff! I hope the next few days will bring us some sort of miracle!

February 24, 1982

I did not see Dan today until late afternoon. This morning they delivered the commode I arranged to borrow from the lodge. A friend sent her cleaning woman over to help me in preparation for Dan's homecoming. We picked up all the small rugs and packed them away.

Yesterday, they removed Dan's catheter and for the first time showed him how to partially dress while still in bed.

He called me several times during the day with the aid of a nurse. He still cannot manage phone dialing with one hand and he has regained only minimal use of his left hand. The droop has left his mouth and eye, however, and his vision seems to have cleared, but there is still some problem with coordination. He seemed disturbed and ill-at-ease without me, even though I had explained to him what I was doing and that I could not be there with him until evening.

We had dinner together at the hospital and parted on a happy, though apprehensive note. *God help us! He's coming home tomorrow.*

Phase 5: Homecoming!

February 25, 1982

I awakened with a feeling of excitement, tempered by anxiety. I am still uncertain as to Dan's condition and more than a little fearful that I will not be able to cope with whatever situation might arise. I went to the hospital as usual about 8 A.M. and waited while Dan had his bath and shave, then helped him to dress, a feat he has only partially mastered.

Our ambuvan driver came by at 9:30 A.M. to take us for the last treatment. Dan was in good spirits at the clinic. He looked much brighter, more energetic and alert, and he was enthused about going home. Before the driver left us, he gave us each a tight hug and there were tears in his eyes. He has been with us every day of radiation, a series that started on February 4.

I had arranged for a close friend to follow Dan and me home in the car to see that he got safely into the house. I brought the car around and closely observed the way the nurse assisted Dan from the wheelchair to his walker and from the walker into the car seat. I tried to fix the image firmly in my mind, to reverse the procedure when we got home.

We were blessed with a warm, sunny day and he thoroughly enjoyed the drive after his four-week stay in the hospital. With help, he alighted from the car, made his way slowly up the short path with his walker, then up the two low steps with the newly installed railing into the house.

Dan sat in a chair while I fixed lunch. A little later he went to bed for a nap, but he was up again for dinner and a visit with our cat, Red. I was concerned that Red would get in front of Dan with his walker and trip him, but with the instinct that pets seem to have, he kept out of the way. Finally at home in his own bed, Dan slept.

March 10, 1982

After a sleepless night, we were both tired. Dan did some of his exercises but spent most of the day napping in bed. He complained that his side hurt. He took some pain medicine and went to bed for the night before 10, but in less than an hour, he was up and thrashing about. He was more upset than I have ever seen him. We went into the family room and I made some hot chocolate.

We sat and talked quietly of his fears. Death. Finances. The ending of his sick leave. His job. For the first time, the word "death" hung between us in the air. I felt a sudden chill. He has always been so confident. So full of faith. I have tried to put any doubts as to his recovery from my mind. He is too young. Too vital. He is too interested in life and has too many things he wants to do. Yet there it was. We both believe in the hereafter. Is it death itself, or the process of dying that makes him fearful? He has always been so strong, one who could cope with any trial or disappointment. Does he now perceive that he just might not get well? If so, what awaits him?

We have always been so close, but this is between him and his Maker. All I can do is to reassure. What if I were the one to go through what he has gone through? And what he is still facing? Would I be all that sure of the future? I have never met a person who is as kind, as compassionate, as gentle. I might doubt my own worthiness to enter the Kingdom of Heaven. I have no doubts about his.

I can allay his concerns about finances. "You still have six months of paid sick leave," I reminded him. "After that, your long-term disability benefits will commence. Then there will be Social Security disability, and ultimately, retirement pay.

"Remember," I continued, "we cut our income in half when I quit my job in 1973 and we have managed very well. We can do it again. Don't worry about money. Concentrate your energy on getting well."

We returned to bed but slept fitfully.

■ ■ ■

Dan had now been home from the hospital for two weeks. It had been a time of ups and downs, of encouragement and discouragement, certainly enough to try the patience of Job and to make anyone depressed.

Having been on the catheter for four weeks, he had to completely retrain his bladder. This involved numerous accidents. I covered our mattress with a plastic garbage bag and was using Chux waterproof pads on his side of the bed for protection, but there was still additional laundry. This concerned him.

We were desperately afraid of his falling, although the therapists had told us not to panic if he did. They had instructed us that, if he fell, he should stay where he was until calm, then crawl over to a bed or chair and pull himself up. That would be fine, I thought, if his bones were not so damaged and frail from the cancer and the radiation. The radiologist had shown me the last bone scan of Dan's entire body, and while I had seen the extent of the damage, I assumed that his body was renewing itself. He did fall a couple of times, but apparently without harm.

The visiting nurse came to check Dan and to assist him with his shower. We rejoiced with each weight gain and each improvement in blood pressure. The physical therapist demonstrated exercises to strengthen his body. We did them together.

I bought him jogging suits. They were warm and comfortable, easy for him to get into and made him feel properly dressed. This boosted his ego. Being in pajamas and robe a made him feel like an invalid.

We had a social life, even though confined to home. Some of the employees he had supervised at work came to visit regularly. They kept him up-to-date on the activities at the office and in their personal lives. They seemed to miss him as much as he missed being at work. Other friends came almost daily. Of course, all visits were brief but much enjoyed.

There were, however, friends who shunned us, staying away as if the disease were contagious. On Dan's last day at work, he had appeared strong and virile. He had worked daily with few absences and it was not until he had been unable to return to the office on December 17 that his health problems became general knowledge. Now, in this short time, he moved slowly and with the aid of a walker. His golfing partners could not cope with this change. They came only once, stayed just a few minutes. They could not even hide their expressions of shock and dismay at seeing Dan so thin and weak. While we were disappointed, we well understood the cancer phobia. Dan's own mother suffered from it. And with some of his male friends, we could almost sense their feeling of "there but for the grace of God, go I." As if to compensate, those who did stay with us became more close and caring.

But while these visits and the demands of daily living filled our daylight hours, the nights were a problem. Dan experienced hallucinations, nightmares and occasional disorientation. Reactions to the medicines? Or had there been some brain damage? I dared not admit this fear, even to myself. The doctor suggested reducing the Decadron to one-half tablet daily to be taken in the morning. The sweats resumed. He could not sleep. Chlordiazepoxide was prescribed. Dan would sleep in fifteen-minute snatches and seem to think he had slept a long time. He complained of chest pain. Troubled now with diarrhea, he started taking Lomotil.

The nightmares continued and the sleeping pill did not help. He developed a fixation about the bladder problem. If the nurses at the hospital had gradually weaned Dan off the use of the catheter instead of just leaving it in for four weeks and abruptly removing it the day before discharge, this problem could have been avoided. I was angry at myself for not having anticipated this reaction so that we could have enlisted their aid before he left the hospital. They would have known the proper procedure.

Tired from the sleepless nights, Dan rested in bed with the cat alongside much of each day. At first I tried to work while they slept, but I, too, was getting tired. I finally started napping with the two of them.

He developed pain in his shoulder from the exercises and from the continued use of the walker. He longed for the day when he could progress to a cane. He worked furiously at his exercises, reaching toward that goal.

Still his sense of concern, his fears of death and of finances, which he had so recently expressed for the very first time, hung in the air between us. During one of our minister's daily visits, Dan told him he was having trouble praying. The pastor brought some books he felt would help and assured Dan that was one of the problems man had experienced in times of stress since the beginning of time. I could not believe that Dan would ever think that God was punishing him, but as a lifelong Christian, being unable to communicate in prayer was obviously painful.

All through these many months, I had marveled at Dan's display of confidence. Did he keep up an act to help me? I didn't think so. We had been much too open with each other through the years. He so desperately wanted to be well and strong again. He had evidenced no anger at being struck with this devastating illness, placed no blame. Now that his fears finally surfaced, I felt I was the one who must keep a positive outlook.

As we struggled with matters of the spirit, we also battled the demons attacking Dan's body. Mylanta was added to his list of medications to help him retain his other medicines—the Dilantin, phenobarbital and Decadron. Though we kept his left leg bandaged and massaged it regularly, the swelling continued. So did the night-mares, which interrupted our sleep.

March 14, 1982

Our wedding anniversary! Twenty-nine great years!

Mom called early this morning to wish us a happy anniversary.

I didn't buy a card for Dan. I knew it would only make him feel sad that he was unable to do any shopping for me this year. He was very upbeat today, however. He talked about how lucky we were to be together and to be overcoming our problems. He said there would be plenty of time for us to celebrate later. He even felt strong enough to stay alone while I went to church. Of course, the cordless telephone gives him a sense of security. Still, this is a milestone and cause enough for celebration!

March 15, 1982

Today we had a full day of doctors' appointments, the first since Dan was released from the hospital. At 11:45 we saw the radiologist. Dan now weighs 143 pounds. Down a little, but still holding well. The doctor suggested that he take the Mylanta after each meal and before bedtime. He explained that the Decadron can cause internal bleeding. He warned, however, that the Mylanta might cause loose stools, but if so, other antacids are available. He then sent us for blood tests.

The next appointment was at 12:30 with the neurologist. The offices are near each other and we made the appointments close together so that Dan would have as little walking and as short a time away from home as possible. He is still very weak.

As we made our rounds, we commented on how doctors' offices are not constructed or arranged with any thought of their patients. This new medical building was built in the center of a block, sur-rounded by a parking lot, but even the disabled parking spots are quite some distance from the entrance. I let Dan out in front of the door, then parked. A ramp led to the elevated first floor and it seemed steep to me. I saw that Dan also had difficulty negotiating it with his walker. We stopped at the lab on the first floor for the blood tests.

The neurologist's office was on the second floor of this multistoried building which had been built around an atrium. Over a highly-polished, irregular tile floor, we made our way to the elevator and exited on the second floor, continuing down the hall to the doctor's office. I counted 210 steps! Dan was very tired. However, good news awaited us. The doctor said the leg swelling is not caused by the veins since there is no pain. We are to tell the physical therapist to concentrate on exercises for this leg. He instructed us to exercise without the bandage and also to remove the bandage whenever the foot is elevated, which should be at all times except when in use. We should do lots of massage, rubbing back toward the heart. He reduced the phenobarbital to 2 grains from 3, and told us to call him in a week.

We had a very good night. The best in weeks!

■ ■ ■

I needed my rest, too. There were constant bills to pay and insurance forms to complete to get reimbursement from our medical insurance. We completed assignments for the larger bills so that the insurance company would pay its share and we would then make up the balance. Though I transferred funds from savings to checking, the bills were taking their tolls and since the bulk of the expenses would be paid by our insurance, we felt the insurance should pay first and let us conserve our resources.

Our federal and state income taxes had to be figured and the forms completed. This was a task we had always done together. Now I completed them while Dan rested.

I pored over the forms I had picked up from the Medi-Cal office and coordinated their information with that from the Veterans Administration. Dan's mother received a small pension from that agency, and one agency always affects another. I was either on the phone or in our office filling out forms for hours at a time.

I packed up all of my mother-in-law's financial records to home with Dan's brother. He had agreed to take over her business affairs now. We had done it for more than eighteen years.

Since Dan was not yet in physical condition to take care of our personal affairs, I drafted a letter of instructions for my sister, his brother and a friend who was to be executor of our estates, setting forth the information they would need if anything happened to me during this period. Someone would have to know where our bank accounts were, the safety deposit box, etc. But as we made these preparations, we became increasingly hopeful that such measures were only precautionary and would never be needed. Reducing the dosage of phenobarbital had eliminated Dan's nightmares and he was much brighter and more alert. With the more restful nights, he was also becoming stronger.

As he improved, the therapist brought us more good news! She thought Dan could now start using a cane instead of the walker. After we were both instructed in its proper use, we started taking short walks twice a day around our cul-de-sac. With the fresh air and exercise and his renewed confidence, Dan's nights were no longer filled with nightmares. He slept better and for longer periods of time. There was no more talk of fears!

Then one night, I was awakened by tremors in his foot. He didn't feel them. I phoned the neurologist. He said to increase the phenobarbital to 2½ grains daily. I discovered I might have been giving Dan the wrong dosage. The bottles of full-grain tablets and half-grain tablets were side by side. If I had given him the wrong pills, he was receiving only half the prescribed amount. The tremors stopped, or at least it seemed so to me. I wondered if they were really gone or if I was just so tired I didn't feel them.

Still, we were almost back to a normal life. I visited Dan's mother regularly and occasionally he rode over with me but stayed in the car. [Not yet ready for rejection?] His brother came out on another business trip and spent a few days with us. It was a time of celebration. He was delighted to see Dan doing so well, and, with his support, both Dan and I felt confident to venture farther than we had thus far. Instead of his usual jogging suits, Dan dressed in slacks and a colorful sweater. He donned a favorite golf cap to cover his sparse hair which had not yet fully grown out. The three of us took care of the necessary business; we picked out a new recliner for Dan and treated ourselves to meals at two favorite restaurants. By the time Charles left, we were all sharing a more positive outlook. We really would overcome!

Dan continued to use his cane exclusively, and we assumed that the change from walker to cane explained the "charley horse" and the sore shoulder he was experiencing. His family physician gave him Naprosyn which relieved the pain. Then the tremors reappeared. I started feeling them nightly. I awakened to every movement, then lay still, dreading another and hoping upon hope it would not materialize. I was afraid of another full seizure. We were instructed to increase the phenobarbital to 3 grains. The nightmares returned, but he could not do without the higher dosage. Still, Dan's strength appeared to improve daily. He was up for longer periods of time, took his walks with me and read.

April 4, 1982

Palm Sunday dawned warm and sunny. After I returned from church, Dan joined me in the car and we drove through the wine country. I needed pictures for an article I'm writing and he felt strong enough to go for a ride. I cannot express the joy and pleasure we both felt at such an outing. Along the way we talked together into the tape recorder, describing the road shaded by ancient oak trees, bearded with moss and mistletoe, the barns, the old country church, the setting that makes the wine country so inviting.

When we got to the winery, I asked the owner if I could drive up to the door, as we were the only visitors at the moment. Dan went into the winery, sat down on a keg and visited while I took my pictures. The warmth of the sun was as nothing compared to the warmth in my heart at having him with me in the car, enjoying the fresh air, the beauty of another spring.

This was our longest drive since he left his work in December and we were gone from home for several hours, yet he did not seem to tire or experience any added pain. A good omen, as we approach Eastertime. We vowed to take many such drives from now on.

Thank.you, dear Lord, for this very special day!

April 8, 1982

Maundy Thursday, and our church was holding Communion Service at 7 P.M. Dan had not been to church for several months, and although he had visits from the minister almost daily, it was not the same. He missed the Communion, the church environment and the fellowship. He thought he was strong enough to attend. I was elated at his decision. I tried to convince him to take his walker, but he insisted the cane was sufficient.

I parked the car directly in front of the church; still it was several steps into the building where we sat in a back pew near the door. We planned to leave quietly as soon as we had been served.

During this special Communion Service, all who wish to go are taken into an *Upper Room,* twelve at a time, where the minister conducts a brief service in much the same manner as Jesus and the Disciples did in that *Upper Room* so many years ago. The room is lighted only by oil lamps. Silver bowls of herbs of Biblical days, hyssop and myrrh, are on the table and the wine is drunk from a silver chalice. We have always enjoyed this impressive service. This year, however, Dan was unable to climb the stairs and so we waited for Communion to be served in the Sanctuary. This was not done until the *Upper Room* service was completed and in the interim, the assistant minister read scriptures and the organist played.

Usually Communion is served starting at the rear of the church and moving forward. This year they happened to start at the front. So we waited. And waited. I wanted to slip down, talk with the assistant, explain Dan's condition and get served, but he wouldn't let me. By the time they finally got to us, we had been sitting on the hard pew for more than an hour and Dan was in considerable pain. When we got home, he took pain medicine and went immediately to bed, but he assured me he was glad he had made the effort. It was very special to him.

■ ■ ■

Even with the increased dosage of phenobarbital, the tremors continued. They occurred only while Dan was asleep. We talked by phone with both the family physician and the neurologist and asked them these questions:

1. *Should the Dilantin level be checked?*
   No. 400 mg. (present dosage) is maximum.
2. *Is there danger of building up to another full seizure?*
   Don't know, but don't worry since he's on so much medication to prevent seizures.
3. *Do the tremors indicate perhaps the radiation did not entirely clear up the tumor?*
   Not necessarily. There could be scarring elsewhere.

4. *What should we do?*
   Don't worry.

Dan took another fall and this time he was concerned. I tried to call the family physician, but he was out of town. I talked with the doctor covering for him, whom we didn't know. He said there had probably been no damage. Later, after considerable pain medicine, Dan developed tightness in his chest and I gave him an Atarax, which has sedative effects. I tried to call the neurologist. He was also out of town and the doctor taking his calls was not available.

Later, when the neurologist saw Dan at his office, he was pleased with his strength and his progress, but when Dan mentioned his painful, restricted left shoulder, he ordered an x-ray, which revealed a new tumor. Radiation started the following day. When Dan told the radiologist about the pain in his right leg, "like a muscle pull," we were instructed to have new x-rays made of both femurs.

I called the lab to make an appointment for the x-rays to be done immediately following Dan's radiation treatment. I explained his weakened condition and that he needed to be saved as much stress, strain and exertion as possible. The lab was near the radiology clinic and by making the appointment I hoped we could take care of both matters within an hour or so.

In the meantime I tried to quell my panic. This cancer seemed to be like a brushfire that kept erupting in new places, just when we thought we had it extinguished. The radiologist had said that only ten or twelve treatments would be needed on the shoulder, but how much could the human body stand and still rebuild itself?

April 15, 1982

Dan rested much of the day in preparation for this new series of radiation and after the treatment, we proceeded to the lab for x-rays. When we arrived, the waiting room was full of people, all ambulatory. Several kids had nothing more than scraped knees. I gave our name to the receptionist and told her we had an appointment. We were instructed to take a seat and wait.

Dan brought his walker today, as he knew he would have considerable walking to do, so his condition should have been obvious.

Fifteen minutes went by. I returned to the desk. "You have to wait your turn."

Another fifteen minutes went by. Dan's face was grey with fatigue and pain. I went back to the desk and reminded her that I had called to make an appointment so that we would not have to wait.

"We can't do that," the receptionist said. "You have to wait your turn like everyone else."

"You don't make appointments?" I was incredulous. "Why wasn't I informed of that when I called?"

She shrugged and turned away.

I looked at Dan. He was so pale and the lines of his misery were clearly etched on his face. She had only to look at him and common sense would have told her to take him first. Nevertheless, we waited. I was furious at her insensitivity.

We waited for almost an hour before the x-rays were taken, then longer until they were checked and we were released to go home.

Dan voiced no protest during the time we waited, but when we got home he said, "Mary, after this is over and you have time to get back on your regular schedule, you must write about this. All the frustrations we have experienced so far. Dealing with so many doctors. Trying to keep them all informed as to what is going on. Knowing who to call when we need help. Perhaps our experiences can help to smooth the way for others."

He was too tired and too miserable to eat. He simply took his medicine and went to bed.

I could cry with frustration! I feel so completely powerless!

■ ■ ■

For the next few days Dan got radiation treatments to his shoulder and both legs. We clung to each other and prayed. This series just *has* to be the last. The cancer must stop here! His left hand, the one which was clenched into a fist so long during his seizure, now gave him pain. His doctor prescribed a new drug, Tolectin. Dan's strength, which had been slowly rebuilding since the January seizure, began to ebb. Radiation treatments were temporarily discontinued so that his body could rest and restore itself. Our frustrations mounted. The medical problems seemed to be slipping beyond our control. And now we faced new pressures from the outside world.

April 28, 1982

Today's mail brought a letter from Dan's employer. He winced as if struck by a blow as he read it, then handed it to me.

The letter was dated April 20. Why had it taken so long to arrive? Then I noticed the name of our street was misspelled. I started reading.

> Due to your extensive absence, I have reviewed your file and I am providing the following, relative to your continued employment with the State Farm Insurance Companies as it relates to your illness benefits. A review of your attendance record reflects . . .

It went on to say that his sick leave would be exhausted on October 30, 1982, and that failure to return to work prior to that date "will result in your termination."

This was our first official communication from his employer, though his immediate supervisor saw us weekly and one of his colleagues visited daily. We were only a few miles from headquarters, yet there was no warning, no phone call, no preparation. It wasn't even a personal letter—just a form letter. After thirty-three years of dedicated service, Dan deserved more consideration than a routine form letter from an assistant personnel manager. It was hardly an appropriate method of communicating such devastating information to a person fighting with every ounce of his strength to get well.

The letter instructed us to immediately apply for Social Security benefits. We were informed that "you may also be eligible for benefits under the disability feature of the retirement plan but that is totally contingent upon receiving a disability award from Social Security."

The letter took us completely by surprise. We knew that Dan had at least four or five months of sick leave remaining and we were holding tight to the hope he would return to work before that time.

Our spirits and morale lagged, though we both tried not to show it. For the first time, in the back of my mind a nagging thought arose, that the company would not let Dan come back, regardless of how much he improved. He was an older employee with a high salary and only a few years [six-plus] remaining until retirement. Will they take advantage of this opportunity to replace him with someone younger for less pay?

As instructed, I immediately called the local Social Security office, gave them the information and was told they would send the necessary forms in the mail.

When his supervisor arrived tonight, Dan showed him the letter. He was furious. He had not been informed that such action was to be taken, either.

Dan couldn't sleep when we went to bed and once again, we got up, fixed hot chocolate and discussed our financial future.

■ ■ ■

The next day we received another letter correcting Dan's termination date to "11:00 A.M., September 16, 1982."

Still a third letter arrived, this one enclosing a set of forms for us to complete.

1. *Attending Physician's Statement of Disability*
    (to be completed by the doctor)
2. *Authorization to Obtain Medical Information,*
    (to be completed in duplicate, one for our doctor and one for the medical reviewer in the home office)
3. *Total and Permanent Disability Report*
4. *Paid Sick Leave Benefit Memorandum of Understanding*

The Social Security forms arrived.

1. *Disability Report SSA 3368 F8* (11-77) (6 pages)
2. *Attending Physician's Statement of Disability*
    We would take this to the family physician.
3. *Authorization to Obtain Medical Information*
    (Required signature and dating only)
4. *Total and Permanent Disability Report*
    (1 page)

I completed them all, thankful for my experience in claims handling for a life insurance company.

Dan developed pain in his elbow which was diagnosed as bursitis. Tolectin was discontinued because it caused headaches and nausea. The doctor recommended applying heat to the sore hip and groin and soaking the left hand in warm water.

Again I inquired about vitamins, minerals, or some type of food supplements. Dan's body had been killed cell by cell by the radiation and he was unable to eat normally. The doctor said, "No. Perhaps an egg milk shake once a day." We could use a multivitamin if we wanted but he didn't think it was necessary.

I took the completed forms to the Social Security office, arriving before the opening time, but still found myself back in line. Since this was my first visit, I did not know about the numbering procedure so by the time I went to the counter to take a number, I was farther back in line. When my turn came, I asked for the claims examiner, as I was carrying with me all the completed forms which we had been furnished, plus the following:

1. Dan's Social Security Statement of Earnings through 1977
2. his W-2 forms for 1978 through 1981
3. certified copy of his birth certificate
4. certified copy of our marriage certificate
5. his Official Notice of Separation from US Naval Service.

I thought I was all set, but the claims examiner looked over these forms, then reached into her drawer and pulled out:

Form SSA-16 F6 (8-78)   4 pages
Form SSA-827 (3-80)   2 pages
Form SSA-795 (2-76)   2 pages

When I asked why these hadn't been sent to us with the others, she merely shrugged and gave the classic response: "Who did you talk to?"

I then learned always to get the full name, exact title, place of employment and phone number of *anyone* I contacted for information.

The paper work and seeing to Dan's care took every waking moment. We had been advised to proceed with a State Disability claim, though we knew he would not be eligible for benefits until his paid sick leave expired, and so I completed "Claim Statement of Employee" for that agency. I wrote to the Veterans Administration asking for forms to submit a claim for Waiver of Premium for Disability under his life insurance policy with them, and sent a similar letter to his private insurer. All these forms were funneled into one small household of only two people. Dan's energies were required simply to survive and to fight his devastating disease. I wanted to concentrate all my time and energy on helping him, yet all these other responsibilities had to be met. The days were not long enough to do all that had to be done. The nights brought little rest.

Dan occasionally complained of a feeling of numbness and lack of control of his legs, but it was temporary. He experienced more tremors, this time during the day so that he was aware of them. His family physician prescribed additional phenobarbital and when that didn't work, I asked about using Valium. The combination kept this under control for a time. When the tremors recurred, I called the neurologist. He said he would discuss treatment with the family physician. This coordination of information and care among doctors was a continuous problem. The neurologist thought the tumor could have spread, but he would need a new scan and more tests to be sure. Since we had an appointment with him on May 11, he advised us just to keep that appointment unless something more happened in the interim.

On his good days, Dan was up and about with his camera taking pictures. His lodge brothers came by and presented him with his Past High Priest's Apron. He stayed up with me later at night, watching television. It was so good just to be together. He could sleep only on his right side so he could no longer hug me up at night, but we continued to sleep like a teaspoon inside a tablespoon.

Other times he complained of weakness, headaches and said his left kneecap "felt funny." It would hardly hold him up. He lost more weight. I wished he were taking vitamins and minerals to supplement his food, which he ate so sparingly, to help replace the cells and tissue destroyed by disease and radiation. Why do doctors not know more about fuel for the body? They seem to be totally ignorant in this area, and I cannot help but think it is of vital importance, especially when one is ill.

There was pain in his right shoulder and throughout his entire pelvic area. It was as if his whole body hurt in one way or another, yet he faithfully did his exercises.

After he was settled for the night, I lay rigid beside him. Always on the alert for the tremors. Hoping and praying they would not materialize.

I continued to visit Dan's mother, as difficult as it was. Though riddled with guilt, I could not forgive her for her denial of Dan. Still, I had to keep contact and see to her care. When Dan's brother had been here, we had discussed the possibility of moving her to a convalescent hospital near him, but we all felt such a traumatic experience for her was not necessary. So I saw her regularly, but I kept my visits brief. I explained Dan's condition to her and asked her to pray with us for his recovery.

May 11, 1982

We had a 9:45 A.M. appointment with the neurologist. Dan prepared the following list of questions to ask each of his doctors:

1. Why don't my legs get stronger with use?
2. When I lift my legs to my chin, the right leg gives me excruciating pain. Why?
3. Why don't I gain weight?
4. When I sit down, practically every bone in my body aches, but I'm comfortable in bed lying on my right side.
5. Should I get a physical therapist back for more exercises?
6. I feel I'm weaker than I should be. What can I do to get stronger?

To his list I added my own:

1. What are the reliable warning signs of a full seizure?
2. Can we get a prescription for Valium for Dan?
3. What can be done about the headaches and nausea?
4. How can we combat the weakness and weight loss?
5. He aches and hurts all over. What can be done to alleviate his pain?

The neurologist responded that numbness or spasms are signs of an impending seizure, but that there are false alarms and the use of phenobarbital and Valium for these symptoms is indicated. He said he would call the family physician and the radiologist. He felt there had been possible metastases to new areas but that at present it would be better to leave everything alone. More x-rays and scans would be needed for further diagnosis and they would be too hard on Dan at this point. We should wait until he was stronger.

We were discouraged but not defeated as we made our way back to the car. "If you were only able to eat more," I persisted. "If we could find some vitamins and minerals you could take that would not have adverse reactions. I'm sure there must be some supplement to help build up your strength."

Dan agreed. "If I could just get to feeling stronger so that I could use my cane again. You know I can't go back to work with a walker."

We proceeded to the radiology clinic for our 11:00 A.M. appointment. The radiologist showed us Dan's x-rays and explained the progressive nature of tumors in bone and bone marrow resulting from prostate cancer. He agreed with the neurologist that at present it would be better to "let sleeping dogs lie." He advised Dan to take as much medicine as he needed to control pain, not to hold back, and to be as active as possible to improve his appetite and his body's utilization of food. He gave us some food supplement samples to try.

It was a sobering interview. I had seen Dan's x-rays before. So had he. Apparently, the reality of the extent of the damage had not fully impressed itself upon us. Also, we believed the body itself was rebuilding. Still, we were encouraged simply by the fact that Dan had been able to withstand the trips to the doctors' offices and the walking and exertion required to make these visits.

Later, his barber came by the house, gave Dan a shampoo and haircut, and he looks almost like his old self. His hair is growing back following the cessation of the radiation treatments, and he was in good spirits as he went to bed.

I wonder, however. *Dear God, will we really win this battle?*

May 13, 1982

I paid my second visit to the Social Security office. Again, I arrived before opening and was number fourteen in line. Our little group stood huddled together in the chill of the foggy morning air.

When the doors opened, we swarmed through, grabbed our numbers from the machine, then took chairs on either side of the lobby. There was a delay in locating Dan's file, but when the examiner scanned the papers I had brought, she said everything appeared to be in order and that we should hear from them in about six weeks. I stopped for groceries, and in all was away from home for about two hours.

Dan called out as soon as he heard me open the door. I ran to the bedroom to find him sitting naked on the edge of the bed, shivering from the cold. Shortly after I had left, he had needed to use the urinal and had stood by the side of the bed supporting himself on his walker, but his emaciated body lost all control. He had tried to clean up as best he could, then sat quietly on the edge of the bed to avoid making a further mess. I threw a blanket around his shoulders, cradled him in my arms and we cried together for several minutes. I knew then I could not leave him alone again.

■ ■ ■

I could no longer deny that he was growing weaker, in spite of the food supplements and new exercises from the therapist. I now assisted him as he got into and out of chairs. I cut up a portion of the egg-crate mattress we had brought home from the hospital and made it into pillows to cushion his aching body. I cried out to him to try harder. "You must stay on your feet so I can take care of you." I coaxed and prodded as if I could will his strength back to him.

Every morning, I crossed off the calendar the events which we had previously penned in for the day . . . golf, dinners, concerts, lodge meetings.

Instead, I got out our booklet that explained the company's fringe benefits program in detail and tried to figure out exactly where we would stand financially in the event Dan would not be able to return to work by 11:00 A.M. September 16, 1982. We had already had one surprise. We had learned that his long term income disability benefit would be almost $200 less per month than we had anticipated because he had not been *actively at work* on January 1, the date of the automatic increase.

There were no dollar amounts quoted in any of the correspondence we had received relating to other benefits, so I studied the handbook and made what I thought were reasonable calculations. My years of work in life insurance were invaluable, as well as my studies for the Life Office Management Institute Fellowship and my International Claims Association degree. I soon had three pages of figures relating to our group medical insurance, group life insurance, group accidental death and dismemberment coverage, and retirement income to discuss with Dan.

He seemed relieved at having some definite figures to think about. If my calculations were correct, we could manage, though the retirement income would be only about 54 percent of what it would have been at age 62 and only 39 percent of the amount available at age 65. There were several pluses. Group medical insurance would continue at the same rate until Medicare took over, and then would act as a supplement. His group life insurance would continue until he was 65, then reduce by one-half and mine would cancel. The group accidental death and dismemberment benefits would cancel, but that was of no great importance. The biggest challenge would be the reduced income, but with care it appeared it would be sufficient to sustain us.

I drafted a letter to the company, asking them to verify my figures and tried not to think of the possibility that Dan might not get well—only that it was taking longer than we had anticipated. Statistics told us that the survival rate for prostate cancer had improved steadily since 1940 and in the past 20 years has increased from 48 percent to about 70 percent.* The odds were in our favor. There was no reason we should not be among the lucky ones.

May 21, 1982

Some time back a good friend and neighbor, a devout Catholic, had asked us if we would be interested in seeing a priest friend of hers who did hands-on healing. We were. Today was the day. She and Father Joe arrived about 10 A.M.

Dan was sitting up in a chair when they came and we talked softly and visited for a time, just getting acquainted. Then we all joined hands and prayed together. Father Joe placed his hand lightly on Dan's head and asked him to relax and meditate.

He gave us some Blessed Salt and a prayer to say as we sprinkled the Blessed Salt around the house. *"Lord Jesus, I ask You to send Your power through this Blessed Salt to cast out and protect us from all evil spirits, persons, things, actions and words."*

He also taught us another prayer. *"In the name of Jesus, through the power of His precious blood and by the authority given to me, I bind the spirit of depression and send it to the feet of Jesus on the Cross. Thank you, Jesus, for taking this away. Please fill the vacuum with your love. Amen."*

With this prayer we are able to give voice to the depression we are both beginning to feel. Recovery is taking so long and there have been so many setbacks. We are both getting very tired.

---

* 71 percent in 1988

Phase 6: The Brushfire Rages On!

May 23, 1982

Dan seemed agitated when he awoke this morning, but he made his way to the kitchen and ate breakfast. At 8:37 A.M. the tremors started. I gave him one phenobarbital and one Valium while he was seated at the counter, then called a neighbor to help me get him back to bed.

I phoned the neurologist but he was out of town. I spoke with the doctor who was covering for him and explained Dan's history. He instructed me to give Dan two more Valium and see if the tremors continued, then more phenobarbital in an hour. He said if that didn't work, we would have to bring him to the hospital for an injection. He suggested a different hospital than the one in which Dan had been treated previously. I didn't know what to do.

I called and talked with the radiologist. He has become more like a friend. I asked him about the change of hospital. He said he thought it was a good idea, as it was a teaching hospital and there were doctors on duty there twenty-four hours a day.

Dan got no relief from the medicine. The tremors grew worse. He was in great pain from the spontaneous and uncontrollable movements. I felt he was on the verge of a full seizure. I called the doctor and an ambulance. At 10:30 A.M. the ambulance arrived to take him to the hospital. I followed in the car.

I was too numb to be frightened and too concerned simply with getting him some relief.

At the hospital emergency room we met the new neurologist. I gave him Dan's medical history as fast as I could, for nothing would be done to help him until the doctor was fully apprised of his condition. It was agonizing to have to stand around talking while Dan suffered.

"Please hurry," I pleaded. "Can't you see the pain he's in?"

The doctor calmly asked, "Is he an alcoholic?"

If our regular attending physician had been available, all this explanation would have been unnecessary. The emergencies always seem to occur on weekends when he is away. It gives me such a helpless feeling.

Finally the tests were made and the injection administered. It was discovered that Dan's Dilantin level was way down. That irritates me. I cannot understand why, four months after his first attack, the doctors cannot get the proper balance of medication to control this condition. Why hasn't the level been checked on a regular basis?

The doctor noticed the MedicAlert bracelet Dan was wearing. I explained the allergies, but I got the distinct impression he gave little credence to my explanation.

The neurologist called the resident physician on duty and suggested that Dan be admitted to Intensive Care. Once again I went through the explanation of Dan's complete medical history. (Who does this for patients who have no family?)

The seizures stopped by 2 P.M., but Dan was exhausted from the movement of the tremors and from the pain. He is being kept in Intensive Care Unit overnight. I know he is safe and is being constantly attended to. That, at least, is comforting. Now I can rest, too.

May 24, 1982

When I arrived at the hospital this morning, Dan was seated in a chair eating a bowl of oatmeal. His movements were awkward as the seizure has once again affected his entire left side. His left hand was clenched into a fist and he had very little use of it. By the way he held his head, I knew that his vision was impaired, too. However, he was more comfortable and was soon released into a two-bed room. I called our family physician and told him what had happened and canceled our appointment with the visiting physical therapist.

Dan spent the day resting and we talked about getting busy once again with the physical therapist to repair the damage done by this latest seizure. *Dear God, how much more can he take and still rebuild?*

May 25, 1982

My feeling of hopefulness was short-lived this morning as I arrived at the hospital to find that Dan had suddenly developed a very high fever. He was taken for x-rays, and an intravenous solution of an antibiotic was started.

Even with the fever, Dan was anxious to begin therapy and the hospital physical therapist stopped by to evaluate his condition. However, her mere touch, and any attempt to manipulate the left leg brought him excruciating pain. She said she would return later.

During the afternoon, we had a visit from our regular neurologist. After he spent some time with Dan, he caught up with me in the hall.

"Mrs. Priest, you know he is not going to get any better."

Yes, I had thought about that, but no, I had not accepted it. Dan *had* to get better. He had already been through so much and had fought so hard. It was unthinkable that there should be no reward for such effort.

I stared at the doctor and watched silently as he walked on down the hall toward the exit. I could say nothing.

Regaining my composure, I returned to Dan's room.

Toward evening the family physician stopped by. I left the room with him.

"Mary, you're not going to take him home this time," he said.

Oh God, the pain! I thought I would suffocate. How could this be true? How could I tell Dan? We had always faced up to our problems and discussed them openly. He had a right to know. I wondered if he was thinking of that possibility, too, or, as at the time of the original surgery two years earlier, will I be the one to destroy his hopes?

My mind and stomach churned while I fought the inward battle.

Soon the therapist returned. As she tried once more to exercise the left leg, Dan clenched his teeth in pain. The words did not have to be spoken. He, too, realized we were losing the fight. We stared at each other for a moment, both nodded, and I took him in my arms.

There was no privacy in our two-bed room, but we really had no need to talk of this. Not yet. We simply clung to each other wordlessly. There was much we would have to discuss. But later. Now we both needed time to accept the news, and it was obvious we would have to accept. Dan had fought until he could fight no more. He was exhausted, and only he knew the extent of his pain.

He did, however, remind me once again, "Mary, when this is all over, you must write about our experiences. Perhaps what we have learned can help someone else."

I am numb tonight. I cannot even pray.

May 26, 1982

The resident physician came into our room this morning to discuss with Dan what measures he wished to have taken to continue life. Fortunately, the roommate, a heart patient, was out taking his stroll up and down the hall at the time. This young doctor, still in training, is also easy for us to talk with. Unlike the older doctors who during the months and years have been noncommittal, even evasive, this doctor spoke frankly. He simply asked, "What do you want me to do?"

Dan answered, "If I cannot get relief from this pain, if I cannot get out of this bed, go home, go out to dinner, resume anything near a normal life, then I want nothing done to extend my agony."

"Does that mean," the doctor asked, "that if you develop another high fever, you do not want us to administer antibiotics to try to bring the fever down, but to simply let nature take its course?"

"Yes," Dan replied.

"Do you want to be kept as comfortable as possible, or will you accept a certain level of pain in order to be alert?"

I watched the exchange. In this matter, even I had to be a bystander. It was not my life. It was Dan's, but I share his feeling that quality of life is more important than quantity.

"I want to be alert," he said.

The deal was made. The file was noted. Where did the strength come from? To cope with such a matter so calmly and decisively? Obviously, God was with him.

After work, when a close friend came to the hospital for a visit and to deliver his paycheck, Dan just as calmly explained the situation to him. The friend's eyes glistened with tears as Dan went on to ask him what had happened at the office today.

■ ■ ■

The next day the urologist stopped by and told us of a new drug recently approved for treatment of prostate cancer. He said it was very expensive.

"Will it cure?" Dan asked.

"No. It is only palliative and may extend your time."

"Then I'm not interested," Dan responded. "I do not want life without cure. The way I am now is not living."

A few days later, I received a bill from the urologist addressed to

"The Estate of Daniel H. Priest." Dan and I shared this grim joke.

As soon as we entered this new hospital, the matter of a catheter arose. I fought and won this battle. The nurses thought Dan was incontinent, but they would just bring him the urinal and then leave. I finally convinced them that it was a matter of sight and physical coordination. He simply needed a bit of assistance, and as I was with him from before 8 A.M. until after 8 P.M. and could help him during that time, I did not think it unreasonable for the nurses to check on him and assist him during the night. It was so important to his morale and his sense of independence, as well as eliminating the possibility of the additional discomfort of infection. I insisted that they pin his call button to his gown where he could reach it with his right hand.

I had to continue to fight for Dan's care. I had already noticed the subtle changes which had occurred since his condition worsened and the ultimate diagnosis had been made. I sometimes had to make the rounds of the hospital's second floor several times before I found a nurse to administer his pain medication.

In fact, the doctor actually prescribed his pain medicine every three hours, saying, "Then, perhaps he will get it every four."

Yet I frequently found the nurses sharing jokes with ambulatory patients walking up and down the halls. Both Dan and I experienced the frightening feeling of loss of control. He could not move and I had difficulty getting him help. Why, I wondered, should other patients receive more attention than my dying husband? Is it possible these professionals, these doctors and nurses whose lives are dedicated to the care of people, cannot face death? Do they consider it a personal affront to their abilities and therefore unknowingly shun those who need them most?

But there was no time for introspection.

Dan now experienced pain throughout much of his body. He could not even turn over in bed without aid. I knew it was frightening and frustrating for him to be so dependent, so I stayed constantly by his side all day. One day a friend came by and wanted to stay with Dan for a few minutes to give me a respite, but he became very agitated. For the first time since all this began, he did not want visitors and he did not want me to leave his side. He was going through an internal crisis. I had to find the strength and serenity for us both.

Because of his condition, and for their own convenience, the hospital moved Dan into a private room. This was a godsend to us, as we were living the last days of our lives together and desperately needed the privacy. We shared our daily devotions and prayers with our pastor. In just a few short days, Dan won his battle with his demons and was once more calm and peaceful.

Then we received another shock. I had not realized that in a teaching hospital, residents are rotated to different duty every four weeks. When a new young doctor entered our room and announced he would be caring for Dan now, I freaked out! We had already dealt with seven different physicians—Dan's family physician, the urologist, radiologist, neurologist, and two other doctors who had covered for the family physician and the neurologist when they were out of town, and finally, the resident at the hospital. Doctor Number Eight was more than I could handle. I explained our situation to him and he just smiled. Later the first resident returned and said he would continue caring for us during the remainder of Dan's stay.

Another brief skirmish won.

The radiologist came by the hospital for a visit, though there was no longer anything he could do. I walked down the hall with him as he left and he put his arm around my shoulder and gave it a squeeze. "Mary," he said, "you should never feel that you have let Dan down in any way. No one could have done more for him or been more loyal than you have."

I turned aside to hide the tears. I did not feel that I had done enough for Dan. There should have been some way I could have made him well. Was the stress he shared with me during my working years a factor in his illness? If I had been able to give him children and a different lifestyle, would this disease still have struck? Yet Dan had always seemed perfectly content with our life together. For that I was grateful. He had never failed me. Had I ever failed him?

During this time, we received another letter from Dan's employer confirming the group medical insurance coverage we would have under either disability or early retirement. This information was comforting, even though we both knew that neither disability nor retirement was likely to come into play. He was on sick leave until September 16, 1982 and it was only May.

June 3, 1982

Dan was very agitated when I arrived at the hospital. One look told me why. The night nurse had pinned him into his blankets to keep him covered. Being partially paralyzed, unable to move or turn and pinned down besides, made him feel trapped. I released him from his cocoon and went to the desk to ask that they not restrain him so. Don't they realize how terrifying it is to be helpless?

I assisted him with his breakfast and because of his disturbing night, he was on the verge of going to sleep when a woman I had never seen before entered the room.

"Good news," she said cheerfully. "I have found a place for Dan at . . ." and she mentioned the name of a local convalescent hospital.

I looked at her in disbelief and said the first thing that popped into my head. "I wouldn't put our cat into . . ."

When Dan's mother had her stroke and we wanted to move her near us, we inspected every convalescent hospital and most residential care facilities in the county. The place this woman spoke of was one we would never even consider.

"But," she stammered, "you can't stay here."

I realized she must be the discharge planner.

Once again we were confronted with this unbelievable tenet that a hospital is not the place for a sick person. When did we give up control over the treatment of ourselves and our loved ones? Who has the right to order a dying patient to be moved about from place to place like a piece of dead brush? Why should we not expect to be treated as human beings instead of nuisances? Are dollars to be the only consideration?

We knew the end was near. We had been told that by all the doctors. We had made arrangements so that no heroic measures would be employed to continue Dan's life. All we asked was that he be kept as comfortable as possible until the end came, that he be given the care that any dying human being deserves and that we be left as much privacy and dignity as possible.

I was angry. I could see that Dan was also upset.

"I'm sure your doctor explained to you that you could not stay here much longer," she insisted.

"No. he didn't," I replied.

"Oh," she said. "Well, I'll have to see." And she left the room.

I tried to reassure Dan, but soon the resident entered the room. This time he was not so cordial. Apparently he assumed that we understood we were to be allowed to stay in the acute care hospital only a limited time; then other arrangements would have to be made.

We hadn't. When you're in a life and death struggle, coping with

daily living, with insurance forms, Social Security forms, taking care of
bills and business activities of your own household and keeping in
regular contact with your mother-in-law in a convalescent hospital,
somehow it just does not occur to you that the hospital is not the place
for a sick and dying person. It is a subtlety that had escaped me.

It was clear, however, that something more was expected of us.
We had both thought that Dan's time was so short; that in the
solitude of the private room we would be able to spend our last few
days undisturbed, but with the comfort that he would get the care
he needed. This was not to be.

Dan was dying. We were both trying to accept this fate. We were
trying to squeeze the maximum happiness out of these last few days.
We were making the plans necessitated by this information and
simply trying to make it through each pain-filled, emotionally drain-
ing day.

We talked over our options.

Could I take him home? He was almost totally paralyzed on his
left side and any movement caused him great pain. His vision was
impaired. He was again troubled with constipation, and the skin on
his tailbone and left hip was beginning to break down. If the nurses
did not know how to care for these problems, how could I? As the
end approached, he would need more and more medication. Could
I administer it? Two aides were required to lift him in and out of bed
for his meals and to change his position. Could I find reliable help,
available help to assist me? I assumed the necessary equipment, the
hospital bed, table, etc. would be available on loan from the Cancer
Society. Would it fit into our modest-sized home?

All day long, we turned over these possibilities in our minds and
in our conversation. By night, we were both exhausted. It had been
an unexpected jolt. We decided we would sleep on it and try to sort
it all out tomorrow.

I returned home immediately after having dinner with friends
and once again pored over the pamphlets given to me in February
by the discharge planner at the other hospital.

There were ads for health care services. These were businesses
through which we could hire housekeepers and cooks, companions,
home health aides, licensed practical nurses, licensed vocational
nurses, or registered nurses. I could not visualize how these people
would fit into a care pattern for Dan. Since no one could lift him
alone, assistance would be needed for position changes throughout

the day and night, so essential to keeping him as comfortable as possible and avoiding bedsores. He was already developing these in the hospital. As his condition worsened, would it be possible to adequately control the pain in a home environment? At the hospital and convalescent hospital, registered nurses were always on duty. Obviously, this level of care could not be provided at home. The cost of private duty nursing would be prohibitive and would be only partially covered by insurance for a limited time.

Would people working through these services always show up for work as scheduled? What would we do if they didn't? I would be on duty twenty-four hours a day. Could I hold up under such a strain? Would Dan, in his pain, and I, in my exhaustion, be able to salvage any quality of life in the few remaining days we had?

I agonized over every question. Suddenly the phone rang. It was Dan. An aide had dialed for him. He was upset and depressed.

Did he want me to come back to the hospital?
Yes.

I dressed in old jeans and a shirt and asked a neighbor to drive me. It was after 10 P.M. and I was upset, too.

The aides brought a cot into Dan's room, and so we spent the night. He reached down his good right hand and we clung to each other for comfort. We both prayed he would be taken, that he would not have to face another painful, wrenching move. We prayed together and individually. I was consumed with feelings of inadequacy and guilt. I truly did not feel that I could care for Dan at home, and yet I felt that I *should* be able to. Were my prayers for his release due to selfish motives or out of concern for him?

I quelled my panic as we discussed the possibility of his going home. We both knew he needed nursing care. He was in constant pain and almost helpless. In past emergencies, he had wanted the ambulance and professional help. Would satisfactory help be available from an agency of volunteers, or even from the people who worked through the health care services for pay? Would he feel secure in relying on such people? What would we do if the assigned help failed to show up? Our experience had already taught us that the visiting nurses services were no longer the answer. The nurse had previously come once a week, stayed about an hour, and the charge was $56.00 for each visit. That was more than full-time professional care would cost per day in the convalescent hospital.

We talked softly, discussing our only two options—home care or the convalescent hospital. With our own soul-searching and the nurses' activities, there was little sleep.

Morning found us red-eyed from tears and lack of sleep, but we had made a decision. It was obvious that Dan needed more professional care than I could personally give, and neither of us would feel secure in having part-time help come in from other sources. In his condition, we felt that home care was out of the question.

Would he consider the convalescent hospital in which his mother was being cared for?

Yes.

If he had to go anywhere, that was where he would like to be. At least those surroundings would be familiar. Surely he would be permitted to stay there until the end.

With a sense of relief at having arrived at another decision, I left the hospital about 8 A.M. to go home and get some rest. As I walked down the hall, a nurse called after me. "Mrs. Priest, you are to see the discharge planner before you leave."

I waved an acknowledgment and went on walking down the hall and out the door, where a friend waited to take me home.

When I arrived home, I phoned the discharge planner. I told her of the events of the night and explained that both Dan and I were very upset and very tired. I needed some sleep. As this was Friday and offices would be closed over the weekend, I would find a place for Dan the first of the week. I was adamant. She reluctantly agreed.

I went to bed and slept for a few hours from sheer fatigue from tension.

■ ■ ■

Over the weekend I visited with my niece who is an aide, studying to become a registered nurse. When I told her of Dan's condition, she said she thought we had little time remaining. She explained that many patients throw off their covers shortly before death and that it is important to let them do this. Can it be that they want to leave this world as they arrived? But if my niece knew and understood about this, why didn't the local nurses? After talking with her, I thought perhaps Dan would be spared another painful move.

When his personal physician visited Dan, he said he saw no reason I could not take him home, though he had previously said I would not be able to. "Look," he said, "he's sitting up in the chair eating."

He seemed genuinely surprised when I told him it had taken two aides to lift Dan from the bed into the chair and that it would take two to get him back. Later, Dan shook his head sadly, exclaiming, "I don't think the doctor fully understands the condition my body is in now."

I visited Dan's mother in the convalescent hospital and, since the office was closed, I inquired of a nurse if there were any vacancies. No. Were any expected? No.

I knew I could not postpone Dan's transfer very long, but I put a smile on my face and reassured him. I tried to get some help for his constipation and for the breakdown of his skin. One of the aides rolled up a washcloth and worked it into his clenched left fist. He massaged this hand continuously.

Early Monday morning I made my way to the convalescent hospital. I thought I was composed, but when I was ushered into the office of the Director of Nurses, she took one look at me and said, "Mary, what's the matter?"

"I have to find a place for Dan," I sobbed and broke into a deluge of tears. She held me until I could go on.

She told me there was no vacancy but that they had a man in therapy for a broken bone who should be able to be released near the end of the week. Could I hold the hospital off that long? I would try. She said she would help me. She then asked for the name of Dan's doctor and when I told her, she frowned. "He is difficult to work with," she said.

"I know," I responded, "but there is no point in upsetting Dan further with a change now."

She agreed.

I stopped to see the discharge planner before going in to see Dan.

"Can't you take him home for a few days?" she asked. "And then transfer him to the hospital?"

"No," I said and stared at her in disbelief. How cruel that would be. Cruel to his spirit, but also to his painracked body. Two trips in an ambulance, each several miles. Was there no thought at all to be given to the condition of the patient? His well-being? His comfort or peace of mind?

I asked her to talk with the Director of Nurses at the convalescent hospital and coordinate the plans.

When I returned home late that night, there was another letter from Social Security and a new form: Vocational Report SSA-3369 F6-(5-79), three pages.

All week long, while I cared for Dan, I silently prayed for a call from the convalescent hospital. He had very little appetite. I took care of all his needs, save medication, during the day, and in his almost helpless condition, I became his shield against the world. He enjoyed his visitors, but he wanted me with him, too. He was miserable from impacted bowels, in addition to his other physical problems. I had increasing difficulty getting him the care that he needed. Only later did I realize that the medical community had already written us off. They could not cure Dan. He was going to die. They directed their attention to those they could help. Practical, no doubt, even necessary, but little comfort to those who are still fighting to preserve purpose and dignity in their remaining days. Sometimes I napped in the chair alongside his bed, stirring only as he stirred and needed some attention. And each day, we shared our prayers and our devotions.

And so we existed and we waited. We had to smile and say nothing to well-meaning friends who still insisted, "You can get well if you just have enough faith and keep thinking positive." Such comments fostered our nagging doubts. Perhaps our belief wasn't strong enough. Our minister was a constant source of comfort. He knew and he understood.

I could not face dinner at home alone. At night, I called upon friends to share a late meal with me; sometimes they invited me to their homes and I took along the cordless phone to be in constant touch with the hospital.

Then the news came. The man with the broken arm was being released Thursday morning. Dan could be admitted that day.

Phase 7: Life in the Convalescent Hospital

June 10, 1982

I arrived at the hospital at the usual hour to help Dan with his breakfast, then packed up his personal belongings. I shaved him and eventually an aide came to help with his bath.

The family physician came by and took care of the paper work necessary for the transfer. Once again, his lack of recognition of Dan's condition was apparent. Did Dan want to go with me in the car, or in an ambulance?

The idea of being lifted in and out of a car with the accompanying movement and pain nearly panicked Dan. He gave me a pleading look.

"An ambulance," we both answered at once.

It was arranged. I followed in the car.

At the convalescent hospital, not only was there a private room waiting for us, one very near the nurses' station, but also an old friend. We were able to spend this first day in the care of a woman who had formerly been our company nurse. She had retired, then resumed work at the convalescent hospital. What a blessing she was. She even overstayed her shift to see that we were completely settled in.

I went into the office to pay the first month's bill, a requirement at convalescent hospitals, and then, while Dan was being examined, I returned home to collect some items which would turn the hospital room into a home. I selected a framed photo of Dan with his lodge officers and two watercolors I had painted to hang on the walls. I packed up a couple of sets of his jogging suits with the hope he might be able to wear them on wheelchair rides out onto the patio. I arranged for a neighbor with a station wagon to bring over the only chair in which Dan could sit with any degree of comfort.

When I returned to the hospital I found the nurses who examined Dan were appalled at the condition of his skin. They assured us they would have it healed in no time. (They did.) I also told them about his constipation problem. They would take care of that, too. It seems that at last he will get sufficient care to keep him as comfortable as his condition will allow. I think we both feel a sense of relief; however, there is still the problem of his mother's reluctance to accept his condition. I walked to his mother's room and explained to her that Dan was now living just down the hall. Wouldn't she like to go see him?

She shook her head "no" and started whimpering. Apparently he is still to be rejected. I asked the nurses if they could help us in this situation, but I said nothing to Dan.

I feel a sense of peace tonight, God.

June 14, 1982

When I arrived at the hospital, I could tell Dan was upset, as if he were frightened, a condition I had noted a day or two before.

"What's wrong?" I asked.

"I have to be able to follow the rules and I can't," he replied.

"What rules?"

"I have to be regular with my bowels. I have to get on schedule with my bladder. I have to be able to do all the things they want me to and keep on their schedule."

I thought I understood what the problem was, but I continued questioning. I had to be sure. And as I did, I became more and more angry at the lack of sensitivity at the acute care hospital.

"Why do you have to do all these things, honey? You can't help it if your body refuses to function as you would like."

"It isn't me," he replied. "Unless I can do all these things for myself, or on their schedule" . . . that word again . . .

"Then what?" I prompted.

"I can't stay here." He was almost in tears.

That's just what I thought. He feels he was thrown out of the acute care hospital and now he is afraid he will be thrown out of here. He thought he was on probation.

As soon as he calmed down, I left and talked with the Director of Nurses. I didn't tell her what was wrong, only that I would like for her to come with me and talk to Dan. I knew that for the problem to be given any credence, the information would have to come directly from the patient.

"Connie, what is expected of Dan so far as keeping on schedule with his elimination?" I asked.

"Only that we don't want him to get an impacted bowel, like he had when he first came here."

"And will you and the nurses help him with that?"

"Of course."

I turned to Dan. "See, honey, it's all right. They just want to help to keep you feeling good."

Then he said what I had hoped he would to make her understand. "You'll keep me here even if I can't?"

"Of course," she assured us.

Peace at last. He now feels secure. There will be no more transfers.

■ ■ ■

With Dan now settled in the convalescent hospital where I had more confidence he would get the necessary help with eating and other essential care, my days became somewhat shorter. I did not go to the hospital until about 11:30 A.M., by which time he had had his breakfast and bath. I shaved him when I arrived and stayed the rest of the day, assisting him with his lunch and dinner, returning home about 7:30 P.M. when he was ready to go to sleep.

After the constipation problems were solved and the skin on his tailbone and hip again healed, Dan seemed to feel secure and a sense of peace enveloped us. We spent hours in companionable silence. He dozed in his bed. I napped in a chair close by. His pain was, for the moment, being fairly well controlled by the medication and he was alert and calm when awake. We were able to maintain some quality to our lives.

I took in our Bible and the *Upper Room* and the *Daily Word*, and each day we had our devotions and prayers. The minister came daily. One colleague brought a copy of the beautiful essay of Jesus and the "Footprints in the Sand." Comforting words which were gratefully received.

Before I left him each night, I would lower the side of his bed and he would hug me tight in his strong right arm and kiss me as ardently as a newly-wed lover.

One day I asked him what he had thought about or visualized when he had meditated that morning of Father Joe's visit.

"I saw that I was not going to get well," he responded. There was no bitterness or anger in his voice. It was simply a quiet statement of fact. I was shaken with emotion at his calm acceptance of the ending of his life. He had obviously made peace with his fate. I needed to make peace with mine.

The arrival of my sister from Illinois gave me much-needed support. Dan was also relieved that she was with me. Now he knew I would not be alone during these final days. While she stayed with Dan, I resumed a bit of social life. I attended the annual installation of officers for my Soroptimist club. As a past president, I was asked to present the pin to the new past president and I appreciated being included in the program at the last minute. Everyone asked about Dan. I explained that some people are just too good to be allowed to live long lives and that Dan was one of those. Mine were not the only tears. Occasionally, I participated in one of my writers' workshops.

There was also business for me to attend to. I completed the additional Social Security forms. I phoned the Disability Evaluation Analyst at the State Department of Social Services who handles the medical development and evaluation of Social Security disability claims and learned that they were waiting for reports from two of the doctors and from the hospital. I followed up on those, meantime giving him the latest information on Dan. He said he should soon complete his handling. I also completed the Veterans Administration Form 29-357 and forms for our private life insurance.

I arranged for his barber to come by the hospital and give Dan another haircut. His hair had now completely grown back, thick and black.

I noticed a lump inside my lower right cheek and brought it to my dentist's attention. He made an appointment for me with a friend of his, an oral surgeon, who immediately excised it. The novocaine wore off while he was in the process of putting in the stitches and I very nearly fainted. I'm sure the stress and strain I was under also had something to do with it.

Flowers and cards and gifts arrived every day, as did visitors from far and near. Dan especially enjoyed his fraternity brothers from college days and their reminiscences of old times. He never said a word about his own illness or how he felt.

Several of his coworkers were regulars. He remembered the names of all their children and exhibited interest in them, their work, their families. One young woman who had been on maternity leave when Dan left work stopped by and his first words to her were, "What did you name the baby?" After one of his employee's visits, during which time they had joked and laughed together and talked about the latest gossip from the office, she accompanied me out into the hall, put her arms around me and started to cry. "Mary," she said, "You were so lucky to have had him."

But Dan wasn't gone yet and these, our last days together, were even more precious.

He still was not to have a satisfactory visit from his mother, though a little progress was being made. The first time the nurse wheeled his mother into Dan's room, she said only "Good morning," and immediately wanted to leave. The second time, she stayed about fifteen minutes. Later, they wheeled Dan down to her room where he stayed only briefly, leaving before she became upset. I hoped and prayed she would soon fully accept him and his condition.

I also hoped he would have another visit from his brother. With Charles's naval service, the brothers had seen little of each other as adults, and I wanted them to have some time together before the end. When I phoned Charles and asked him to come, he didn't think it would be possible and sent us a letter to that effect. When I showed the letter to Dan, he said only, "Tell Charles I'm not going to die in the immediate future and for him to come out later when it is more convenient for him."

There was no anger or resentment, but perhaps a trace of sadness. Later, he asked me to bring our cordless phone over to the hospital so that he could talk with Charles. When I explained that it would not work so far from its base, he laughed and said, "Of course not. I wonder what I was thinking."

And after two weeks of apparently holding his own, his condition seemed to deteriorate just a bit.

One morning, as the scent of honeysuckle blossoms seeped through the window and we had completed our daily devotions, Dan lay quietly with his eyes focused somewhere in the distance. Suddenly he asked, "When are we going home?"

My heart stopped for a moment and tears welled up in my eyes. My throat tightened and I did not think I could possibly answer him. Somewhere from the depths came a bit of composure. "Honey," I responded, "remember? We are not going home this time."

"Oh yes, that's right," he sighed and drifted off to sleep.

Later, when he awakened, he called me to his bedside. "I love you too much to hold you to me," he said. "If someone comes along who would take good care of you, go with him."

I did not answer. I could not answer. I just lowered the side of the bed and he put his strong right arm around me and hugged me tightly to his chest.

How did we manage to do this without dissolving into tears? I do not know. I know only that we did and that we hugged our time together as tightly as we hugged each other. Every precious minute, to be savored and stored, and yet we did these things as if we would always be together, and the parting was only until tomorrow.

Footprints in the Sand

One night a man had a dream. He dreamed he was walking across a beach with the Lord. Across the sky flashed scenes from his life. For each scene he noticed two sets of footprints in the sand, one belonging to him, the other to the Lord.

When the last scene of his life flashed before him, he looked back at the footprints in the sand. Then he noticed that many times along the path of his life there was only one set of footprints. He also noticed that it happened at the very lowest and saddest times of his life.

That really bothered him, and he questioned the Lord about it. "Lord, you said that once I decided to follow you, you'd walk with me all the way. But I have noticed that during the most troublesome times in my life there is only one set of footprints. I don't understand why in times when I needed you most you would leave me."

The Lord replied, "My precious, precious child . . . I love you and would never leave you. During your times of trials and suffering, when you see only one set of footprints, it was then that I carried you."

[author unknown]

July 2, 1982

For weeks Dan had eagerly anticipated his birthday and frequently commented, "I don't know why I'm so excited about my birthday this year."

But we did know. It was because it would be his last here with us.

My sister and I arrived at the hospital later than usual, having allowed time for her to put the finishing touches on the tall angel food cake she had baked. Birthday mail had been arriving for several days and he already had a bouquet of pink roses from one of the nurses.

Dan was in his chair eating lunch and the entire hospital staff gathered around him to sing "Happy Birthday" as they lighted the candle on the cupcake which was his dessert. He smiled, blew out the candle and willingly posed for pictures.

As the day progressed, more gifts and cards arrived, along with a fuschia and white basket bouquet, a ceramic planter filled with greenery, a mixed bouquet. One of his colleagues brought a bottle of Dan's favorite gin. His brother sent a cactus arrangement, a nostalgic reminder of their Nevada desert heritage. I gave him a clock for the wall, one with large numbers he could read from his bed.

The day was warm and sunny but a trifle windy. Aides lifted Dan into a wheelchair and about 3 P.M. we went out onto the patio for our party. Dan's mother refused to go with us, but several of Dan's friends from his office came by and we cut the birthday cake, all the while taking pictures of this festive occasion. Dan had so looked forward to this day and he enjoyed it thoroughly, though it left him exhausted.

Returning inside we found his mother in her wheelchair in the hall and we stopped, hoping for a visit. She held his hand briefly, wished him a "happy birthday," then wanted to return to her room. Later my sister took her a piece of the birthday cake.

During the day Dan had eight visitors from his office in addition to my sister and me and the hospital staff. He was very tired. He was up an unusually long period of time for him, perhaps an hour in all. This is the first time he wanted to be outside, but I hope there will be other days like this in the future.

He said it was the best birthday he had ever had.

■ ■ ■

The very next day, he wanted another party. Bobby and I arranged to have dinner with him at the hospital. I asked him if he wanted anything special. "I want a martini served in our Baccarat crystal glasses." He took only a sip or two but thought it was wonderful. I had taken over a couple of TV tables and folding chairs, and the three of us dined in style.

But immediately thereafter, I noticed a change in Dan. He was more subdued, quieter. The anticipation of his birthday had given him a high. Now it was over. What did he have to look forward to? He lost more weight.

He reminded me that this was the year we had planned to take a vacation drive through the South and visit his two elderly aunts whom I had never met. One lived on a farm outside a small town in Tennessee and the other in Arkansas. While I had not met them in person, I did know them. We had corresponded for years, talked together frequently on the phone, and after my mother-in-law's stroke, I had been her correspondent with all the family. Dan and I had planned to attend the Kentucky Derby in Louisville, then rent a car and drive through Kentucky, Tennessee, Arkansas, and return home from St. Louis. He instructed me to make the visits the very next time I went back to the Midwest. We both understood when that next trip would be; it did not have to be said. It would be for his burial in the plot we had purchased years ago at Woodlawn Cemetery in my hometown in Illinois.

I gave him my word.

The medicine he had been taking no longer relieved his pain; still he did not complain, but compressed his lips more tightly together as if to keep it inside, out of view. The Director of Nurses visited him daily. It was she who asked him if he was ready for something stronger. On July 7, he received his first injection of morphine.

The same day his brother Charles and his wife Suzanne arrived. We left the two brothers alone much of the time. They had been separated all of their adult lives. Now they needed to be together. At night, my sister Bobby joined us, and the four of us went out to dinner, a silent, saddened group.

After they left, I sensed another change in Dan. His condition regressed even more. He had been deeply moved by his brother's visit and obviously something passed between them neither had experienced before.

Each Sunday Bobby and I attended church and brushed aside the tears as we heard Dan's name among those for whom prayers were said. We longed for a miracle of healing, but if that was not to be, *please, God, let his suffering be as brief as possible.*

Even here in the convalescent hospital, and with Dan's condition ever more apparent, some visitors would still say, "You can get well. You can lick this, Dan. Just have faith." They did not mean to be cruel; yet such statements *are* cruel. At the beginning of the illness, or even a few months earlier, such remarks would have been appropriate, but now even they should accept the inevitable. A deep, abiding faith was the rope to which we were clinging in this sea of sadness and grief. Any words that insinuate a lack of faith or undermine one's confidence are better left unsaid.

One day Dan lay quietly staring at the ceiling of his room. I could scarcely determine if he was awake or asleep.

"What are you looking at so intently?" I asked. "What do you see?"

"I see a stage," he answered. "And on the stage are all our nieces and nephews."

"And where am I?" I whispered.

"You are in the center of the stage."

"And where are you?"

"I'm watching," he replied, "from someplace far off." And he dozed off to sleep.

There was no place I wanted to be except with Dan, yet my sister informed me he was concerned about my getting on with my life. There was also business for me to handle. Bobby's presence at this time was a blessing. One of us was with Dan all day. Whenever I had things to do, she stayed by his side and wrote beautiful prayers for his release from pain and suffering.

Prayers for Dan

Please Father, erase my brother's fears;
Send Jesus to lead him out of the misery
Into the peace he so richly deserves.
Take him home to your beautiful Land of Glory.

We thank you for the gift of this flower on earth,
For the rich life he had patterned and his dear love;
We ask not for ourselves for we are selfish and want him near,
All-knowing Father, you need him for your kingdom above.

The rose wilts but the thorns continue to destroy.
From the most beautiful flowers you must choose,
Leaving the weeds and thorns to suffer on earth
For this life the eternal beginning is too precious to lose.

Reward this life with the peace we know will come
When brother, husband and son are wrapped safely in your arms.

Fear not, Dan. Reach out and take Christ's hand.
He will lead you across the troubled waters
Out of the misery and pain of this weary land.

Mary's fine, Ellen's fine and so is Charles.
Put your troubles away and reach out your arms.
Jesus will lead you out of this land of strife
To the reward of no more disease, worry and harm.

                    Roberta Woodward (Bobby)

The weather turned very warm. I gave Dan alcohol baths every
few minutes to help to keep him comfortable. He was having difficulty
sleeping. I could well understand why. An elderly woman in a nearby
room had apparently had a stroke and kept yelling—night and day.

Though he was receiving injections for pain, it was essential that
his other medications be continued . . . the Dilantin, phenobarbital
and Mysoline to prevent seizures, and Synalgos, Tylenol and
Phenergan suppositories to aid in control of pain. It was difficult for
him to swallow and keep down the oral medicine. The medicines
were crushed into applesauce and the nurses and I worked with him
with each administration. Cold towels on his head. Small bites. He
ate very little, grew weaker and thinner. His body was rebelling; still
he did not complain.

Each day brought visitors. We wished we had thought to have a
guest book in the room for them to sign. There were so many, we
lost track of who had been there. Dan had visits from his lodge
brothers, his colleagues at work, fraternity brothers and college
chums, friends and neighbors, even his radiologist. The minister
came daily. Dan was happy to see them all, but now the visits were
shorter as his strength and stamina seemed to ebb each day.

I wondered how long it could continue. I talked with the Director of Nurses. "Connie, how long do you think it will be?"

She answered me with a question. "Mary, have you let him go?"

I had not thought of that. No, I guess I had not really let him
go. I did not think it was a direct act that would have to be made on
my part, and yet, perhaps it was. We were so close. Truly one, if any
couple can be. Was I hanging on? Was that affecting Dan's ability to
pass in peace? Was he waiting for some sign from me that it was all
right for him to give up the fight? Questions, always questions.
Where was I supposed to find the answers?

I returned to his room quite shaken. I did not want it to end this way. I wanted him to get well. Reason and logic told me he could not. It was selfish to expect him to continue any longer than necessary.

I was lost in my own misery as I heard Dan talking with someone. As if answering questions. "Yes." "I know." "I will." Yet there was no one in the room with us. I went over to his bed. He was awake and alert. He seemed quite at peace and unafraid. Whose questions had he answered?

I remembered having been with my father when he passed away. How he had done the same. Is there a time, I wondered, before we cross over, when we are a part of both worlds?

Each day I visited his mother and tried to prepare her for Dan's passing.

At home, I found the book he had filled out, like all good Masons, with his final wishes and funeral arrangements, a book he had completed in the 1960s and kept up-to-date, but there was one important question I did not know the answer to. I had to ask.

"Dan, do you want an open or closed casket?" The words would scarcely come out and in my chest there was that familiar feeling of suffocation.

"Closed," he replied, with no show of emotion, but we clung to each other more tightly than ever as I got ready to leave. He had slept soundly and peacefully most of the afternoon, and I left feeling that we had come to yet another plateau. How long would this one last?

I marveled at Dan and his calm acceptance of his fate. No one could possibly set a better example of how to die with dignity. Unlike those who are taken swiftly with heart attacks or accidents, he had every opportunity for bitterness, self-pity, resentment, anger; yet he displayed none of these.

It was obvious that the medications did not control the pain. He suppressed his moans as he was lifted to change positions. I could almost feel the misery with him. Surely there should have been some more effective pain medication available. I longed for his agony to cease.

July 19, 1982

When I arrived at the hospital this morning, Dan seemed a bit stronger. The aide said he had eaten a good breakfast and he had had a bath in the Jacuzzi.

Though by this time they were trying to conserve his strength, he insisted on being up in the chair again for his lunch. He ate well, keeping both food and medicine down. I hugged him tight, but he said, "Don't hover." I realized that perhaps I did have to give him some sign that I could let go.

"Okay," I said.

We did our daily devotions and he joined me in the *Lord's Prayer*. We both settled down for afternoon naps.

About 4 P.M. he started coughing and could not stop. I summoned a nurse. A suction machine was brought into the room to clear the fluid. The shots were given more frequently now as the coughing wracked his body. A humidifier was used to help his breathing. A friend stopped by but Dan was too weak to talk. He quieted for a time, tried a little supper but was unable to eat. The coughing began again.

The Director of Nurses, who had been in San Francisco attending a class all day, dropped by at 7 P.M. and stayed with us until 10 P.M. She thought I should call my sister, which I did. A neighbor boy drove Bobby to the hospital and collapsed into tears when he saw his "Uncle Dan." He wanted to talk with him, but Uncle Dan was not able to talk. I accompanied the boy into the hallway and held him until we were both able to stop crying.

The day's mail had brought a letter from Charles, which Bobby brought with her, a beautiful, moving letter. I read to Dan aloud:

Dear Brother Dan,

Just wanted to send you a note to tell you, Mary and Bobby what a good trip it was to see you all and Ellen. It was mighty tough to say goodbye to you and Mary when the visit ended. It was also so nice to meet Bobby, from whom we got a most appreciated and kind letter today. Please thank her for us.

We all wish things could be different, Dan, but God's will works in various ways, as you appreciate more than most. You are fortunate in having the many good friends you have out there, developed over the years, and well and ably earned through your own friendships and help to them in other circumstances. Their love and visits, I know, mean a lot to you and Mary, even if at this time they have to be monitored and kept brief.

It was also great, from I think all our standpoints, to have Mom visit and hold hands with you.

Words tend to fail at a time like this, except to reiterate our love for you and Mary and for the travail you are experiencing. You have been very brave, both of you. The fact that we all go eventually doesn't end or ease your trauma. However, knowing you have lived a relatively long, and a very meaningful and worthwhile life, means a lot. You have been, and are still, a contributor to this planet and all remember you with love and esteem, for you have been a most kind and good person. Your period of passing on this earth has been for the betterment of mankind, and you leave the world a little better for your stewardship.

No man can ask for a better epitaph than that.

Again, our visit was wonderful from our standpoint, and I gather it was helpful to you and Mary, too, and it gave us a chance to meet Bobby as well. Don't really know what effect it had with Ellen, [their mother], but guess it helped her, too.

Give everyone our love. We bless you all. May God give you peace, respite from pain and His blessing.

Bobby and I stayed the night, taking turns sleeping on the couch in the lobby, so that one of us was with Dan at all times. In the morning she went home to get some rest and a change of clothing. I refused to leave. Dan and I had been in this battle together from the beginning. I would see it through to the end. I knew I would have him only a few hours longer and I wanted to be with him every minute.

The coughing continued. Sometimes more quietly as the medicine took effect, then again more forcefully. I thought of our letters to our senators and wished they could see someone suffer like this. Surely then the laws could be changed to allow for more effective means of dealing with pain. Dan could not eat. They did not lift him from his bed, only turned him and changed his position frequently to keep him as comfortable as possible. I sat there wondering how long this could go on. Not wanting him to suffer longer and not willing to let go.

The family physician came by in the afternoon and asked, "How long has he been like this?"

"Since about 4 P.M. yesterday," I replied.

"Then it is time just to let him go, isn't it?"

"Yes," I whispered.

I did our daily devotions and said our prayers aloud, as usual. The minister came. I was not sure that Dan knew he was there, but I think he did.

Hours dragged by and day turned into night. I prayed by the side of the bed, *My darling, let go and let God take you away from this.* Over and over I repeated the words. They were torn from me, for I did not want to say them. Somehow I felt I must. Did I think about, pray about his death as a release for him, an end to his suffering, or my own? To get off "hold" and on with life? Is there any way to sort this out, to separate the feelings? Are they only human? *Altruistic. Selfish.* The words tumbled about in my consciousness.

A neighbor brought Bobby back in the evening and again we stayed the night.

The nurse whom we had known for so long stayed with us until midnight, though her shift ended at eleven. She stayed to introduce me to a new night nurse, not wanting to leave me with a stranger at this emotional time.

All day Dan had gone without food or drink, wracked by the periodic coughing and labored breathing, relieved only temporarily by each morphine injection.

He had scarcely spoken since the coughing spells began. About 4 A.M. he awoke and the spasms started again. I rolled his bed up a little higher, hoping the change in position would provide some relief.

"Thank you," he said. The last words he was to speak.

The nightmare continued. Aides brought us coffee and Bobby and I took turns in the room, never leaving him alone.

Shortly before noon, the nurses asked us to leave the room so they could turn Dan and put on a fresh gown. We went to the staff room to get a plate of lunch and returned.

Propped up against the pillows, Dan was fresh and clean and almost comfortable-looking, save for the shallow breathing and the pulsing beats of his heart which were so strong they shook the bed. Suddenly, the shaking stopped. There was one slight flutter and he was gone. He closed his eyes in sleep and the pain and suffering left his face for the first time in months. With his hair now grown back, full and black, he looked like the handsome young man with whom I had shared the marriage ceremony only twenty-nine years before.

I could not believe his eyes were closed in death. Surely he was only sleeping. His left hand, clenched into a fist for weeks and weeks, was relaxed and normal. I thought of his Grandpa Goodrich's admonition. Yes, those beautiful blue eyes did break some girl's heart, but only because they closed too soon.

I leaned over him, tears streaming down my face. I would not have him back to suffer, but, oh, I did not want him to die! Why did he have to be one of those who do not get well? I bathed his face and brushed his hair, all the while assuring him that I would be all right, that I would look after his mother, that I would love him forever. I kissed him and held his hand as his life flowed out.

In a few moments, the nurse insisted that I leave. "You're still alive, Mary," she said. "You've got to go on."

For the first time, I was forced to go away and leave him. I did not think I could do it.

I went into the office and called the mortuary. The mortician is a friend, but even so, my composure was about to disintegrate when her voice came on the line. All I could say was, "Patsy, I need you," and I had to give the phone to the nurse to complete the arrangements.

I returned to the room and Bobby and I started collecting Dan's things to take home. The jogging suits he had never worn. He had never been sufficiently free from pain, nor had sufficient stamina, to be dressed in anything other than gown and robe, and except for his birthday, he had not left his room. Several times, we were interrupted by soft knocks at the door. Nurses, aides and staff came in shyly to ask, "Mrs. Priest, may I pay my respects to Mr. Priest?" They would go to his bed, touch his hand gently, turn to me and say, "I'm so sorry. He was such a wonderful man."

Dan had asked that we leave the clock in the room. I also left the two watercolors, hoping they might brighten someone else's stay.

Soon we had gathered everything. Everything but my beloved Dan whom I had to leave lying in the bed. They say a heart cannot break. That's not true. I could feel mine rending into pieces as I walked from the room.

Dan's suffering ended at 11:55 A.M., July 21, 1982. Would mine ever end? He showed us how to die with dignity. *Dear God, may I now exhibit some of that same courage as I face my life alone.*

Phase 8: A Celebration of Life

I HAD NO FEELING INSIDE, only emptiness. It was as if I were dead, too, as I automatically went through the motions of all that now had to be done. It was a routine learned long ago and performed by rote. I had been programmed from childhood to go through the death rites. In the small farm community where I was raised, children were not sheltered from the facts of life. Funeral attendance, taking food to bereaved families, all these were a part of my heritage, for which I was thankful.

I made the phone calls to minister, family and friends. Since Charles had been here only two weeks earlier, I did not expect him to return for the funeral, but he assured me that he and Suzanne wanted to come.

I sat down at my typewriter to prepare Dan's obituary. How could his lifetime of love and service be reduced to a few lines of print? There was no way. Written words would only skim the surface. His true obituary would be lived out in the lives of all who had known him.

I selected his burial clothing, a favorite suit and tie, a crisp white shirt and his Masonic apron. My sister and I took them to the funeral home. I then chose a deep brown mahogany casket. We liked things plain and natural. The minister met us. We completed the funeral arrangements, to be carried out according to Dan's written instructions. The service would be simple—a message from our pastor who had shared each day of these last trying months with us and the traditional Masonic funeral service which Dan himself had given many times.

At the florist shop we ordered our memorials, then returned to the funeral home to see Dan. He looked as if he had stepped out of our wedding picture. All evidence of pain and suffering had vanished from his face when life passed from him. Such peace and tranquility. I could scarcely believe he was gone.

Flowers had already arrived and by the evening visitation period, they filled the room.

I was so grateful for my sister's company. Her love and support helped to get me through the pain-filled days. With friends and neighbors, she planned the Celebration of Life which would follow the funeral.

July 23, 1982

Never in my worst nightmares had I dreamed of having to attend my husband's funeral so early in our lives. Even though my father died at fifty-six, I felt he had had a complete life. My sister provided him with grandchildren and I gave him an excuse to travel. He had enjoyed farming from childhood and death claimed him before he had to give up his occupation. He was completely mobile and active until he went into the hospital for the surgery which, with its complications, together with the cancer, took his life in only twelve days. Somehow it seemed Dan had died too young. He was so youthful in appearance, so energetic, so full of plans for the future. He would have enjoyed retirement. But now, of course, he would never retire. I resented this awful disease which had struck him down—a disease that attacks people in the prime of life and one that has reached such epidemic proportions.

Somehow, I had to get through this day.

Charles and Suzanne arrived. We all lunched on the food that neighbors had brought, then showered and dressed and returned to the funeral home for the 2 P.M. service.

I told myself that no one attends funerals anymore, but the parlor filled rapidly. Chairs were brought in and set up in the rear and in the adjoining hallway. I was overwhelmed at this outpouring of love and support from friends, neighbors, colleagues who came to pay their respects. More than two hundred in all. Dan's mother was brought in her wheelchair and after the service, the casket was opened briefly so that she could see Dan. She seemed to understand.

About fifty people returned with us to the house for a celebration of Dan's life. The white damask cloth Dan had purchased in China so many years ago covered the dining room table now burgeoning with food. I had taken a yellow rose from the casket blanket and placed it by Dan's picture on the coffee table.

These, our family and closest friends, filled the rooms of the house he had helped to design and spilled out onto the patio, whose 2,200 bricks had been personally laid by Dan and me after our home was completed. I moved from group to group, listening to the stories and the memories we all shared. No, Dan would not be forgotten. We toasted his life and the influence he had had on us all. Everyone stayed and stayed, reluctant to depart, as if in so doing, they had to let go of this precious friendship.

■ ■ ■

The four of us shared a family weekend as we consoled each other and tried to rest, yet each was lost in his own grief. Sunday, Charles and Suzanne returned to their home in Virginia.

It was not yet over. There was still the burial in Woodlawn Cemetery in Clinton, Illinois. Dan and I had bought our plots there in 1973, the summer after his chest surgery. We had talked about where we wanted to be buried. With no children, it was a difficult decision to make. His father was buried in Reno and his mother would be buried there, too, but Nevada was where they spent most of their lives. Dan had lived in Nevada until he left for college. His ties there had long since been broken. His brother would be buried in Arlington. We had decided on Woodlawn in my hometown of Clinton, Illinois, where there were five generations of my family already at rest. We purchased lots only a few steps from where my father, grandparents, aunt and uncle were buried—on a gentle slope, facing the rising sun.

Arrangements for the Clinton rites were made by phone, an evening visitation followed by graveside services conducted by my sister's minister. Then we mounted the plane for home.

A feeling of numbness settled over me, isolating me even from my sister and I kept my silence as the miles went by, on the ground and in the air.

I had been gone from my hometown since 1943 and from Illinois since 1946, so I was scarcely a part of the evening visitation at the Clinton mortuary. These were Mom's and Bobby's friends. Naturally their conversations were of local matters. I felt so alone, a bystander, as the ritual played out before me. Since the casket was to remain closed, I had brought along a framed picture of Dan which was displayed on a small table. From his photo, he smiled at me reassuringly.

July 30, 1982

At 2 P.M., wearing the same dress I had worn to the funeral on the 23rd, I joined Mom and Bobby, nieces and nephews at the funeral home where we accompanied Dan's body for the short drive to Woodlawn Cemetery. There I was pleasantly surprised to see among the gathering of friends and relatives Dan's former colleagues who were now assigned to the nearby home office. More evidence of the high regard in which he was held.

The service was brief and beautiful. I gazed out beyond the open grave to the field of deep green corn maturing on the other side of the fence and was reminded once more of the never-ending cycle of life and growth.

Soon it was time to return to my mother's house for a family dinner. I hoped that having lost Dad so many years ago, she would understand how I felt. That I needed to talk about Dan, but every time I started, she changed the subject. I was hurt, but I thought, perhaps talking about Dan brought back sad memories of Dad, and so I stopped trying.

Aunt Helen was even joyful. "Isn't it wonderful!" she said. "Dan is now with his Father in heaven!"

My reply was as sharp as the pain I felt inside.

"Yes, Aunt Helen, it is wonderful that his suffering is over and that he is with his Father, but it is a tragedy that a person so young, so vital, who so loved life and was so looking forward to the future had to be stricken in the first place. He had everything to live for, while there are millions of elderly infirm who have nothing to live for. The tragedy is living too long, or dying too soon."

■ ■ ■

Next morning I selected a monument for Dan's grave: a small dark grey granite which had been hand-polished by Amish craftsmen in Pennsylvania. The dealer also took care of the paperwork for me for the bronze veteran's marker.

Now it was time to visit the aunts.

My sister agreed to accompany me. The first day we drove to Louisville, Kentucky, where we stayed the night and visited Kentucky Horse Park next morning. While there, I took pictures, collected pamphlets, recorded the tour guide's spiel. Perhaps an article would result from this. Was this the start of the healing process? Or was I still being selfish to be thinking of such an idea at a time like this?

We continued to Knoxville where we stayed with Dan's cousin for two days and attended the World's Fair. Again I felt the hurt of having Dan ignored. My sister and Dan's cousin, both avid talkers, chattered about everything, but when I mentioned anything about

Dan or our life together, they changed the subject. Finally, I said, "You are both acting as if he never existed."

His cousin looked at me, somewhat surprised. "Well, Mary, you can't expect us to feel about it as you do."

No, of course not, I thought, but to ignore his existence is cruel. I thought she would understand, having been widowed, too; but, like Mom, was it so long ago that the wounds had healed and the scars were no longer painful, or, having endured such a loss, they feel everyone should just take it in stride.

I was tired of the way people reacted to this tragedy. The people who said, "I know just how you feel. I lost my mother/father to cancer."

No, they didn't know how *I* felt. Mothers are mothers. Fathers are fathers, and no one could have loved a father more than I loved mine, but spouses are different. Even spouses engender different responses. There are no relationships between any two people that are the same. No one can ever truly know how another person feels about anything.

If someone would have only said, "I know you must feel a great deal of pain, anguish . . . Is there anything I can do?" Or simply, "I'm so sorry."

Most of all, I needed a hug.

Another day's drive brought us to the small village of Hurricane Mills, Tennessee, where Aunt Sophie lived with her daughter Jane and son-in-law on a farm. Nearby was the small town of Waverly where Dan's mother had been born and raised. We toured the family homestead and the cemetery. Dear Aunt Sophie. From the wisdom of her ninety years, and recently suffering a recurrence of the cancer to which she had lost a breast some forty years earlier, she hugged me tight and said, "Mary, I kept praying that the Lord would take me, not Dan."

The warmth of family, the quiet of the Tennessee farm, the watermelon feast by the light of fireflies brought some sense of peace.

On to Pine Bluff, Arkansas where Aunt Dean lived in an all-care retirement facility, though she was as full of life as a teenager, slowed down only by the arthritis she tried to ignore. From Aunt Dean, there was also a word of comfort. "Mary, there is only one positive thing to come out of this experience. That is the knowledge that you have already experienced the worst thing in life that can happen to you."

Yes, I thought, *there will never be a year as happy as those of the past, nor any as painful as the one I have just been through.*

When we returned to Clinton, I visited the cemetery and found that the stone had been set in place. The earth was still bare, but I knew that seed would be sown just before the fall rains, and that on my next visit the grass would be green and Dan's grave would blend in with all those lovely ones surrounding it on the gentle hillside. I prayed over his grave and bade him farewell. It was time to go home.

Friends met me at the airport. I had made the trip to Illinois many times by myself over the years, both on business and pleasure, but for the first time in twenty-nine years, Dan would not be at home to greet me. I was coming home to an empty house.

I treated them to lunch en route home, delaying my arrival as long as possible. I was anxious to put my life together, yet hesitant to start. I knew I would be busy over the next few months taking care of business. After that was done, what then? Dan wanted me to write our story, the events of the past two years. Could I?

The big red cat was glad to see me but scolded me for my long absence. I hoped he would stay with me at night, sleep on top of the bed, as he had with Dan, but he knew something was wrong. Someone was missing. He retired to his bed in the garage.

August 24, 1982

I steeled myself for the trip to the hospital to visit Dan's mother this morning. I had been gone three weeks. How would she greet me? I felt the pain that Dan—vital, youthful, energetic Dan—was gone. Ellen, some four-and-a-half years after her disabling stroke, remained. Do I resent her? I really don't know. In the past few months I have. Now she is a living link to him. That somehow makes her more precious to me and eases the pain.

She was sitting in her wheelchair near the front window when I entered. Her speech, temporarily uncluttered from the effects of the stroke, was clear and firm as she asked, "Where's Dan?"

I caught my breath, that familiar feeling of suffocation enveloping my chest. I hugged her as I answered, "Remember, Ellen, Dan's gone. Remember? You went to his funeral."

"Oh, yes."

■　■　■

I returned to an unbelievable stack of mail and once again I was overwhelmed at the outpouring of love and sympathy for Dan and for me. Over a hundred cards and letters indicated how special he was to so many people. Memorial contributions to the Cancer Society, his lodge and numerous charities must have totaled hundreds of dollars. I read and reread the beautiful cards and letters.

The folks at the convalescent hospital sent me a lovely hibiscus plant in full bloom. The board of directors of the country club sent an attractive dried arrangement. Remembrances came from people I would never have anticipated.

But there were the minuses. The acute care hospital where Dan had last been a patient called to ask me how he was. The young caller did not even seem nonplussed when I replied, "He is dead." Such a follow-up program is commendable; however, I feel that some discretion should be used. Files, such as Dan's, which had been coded for no treatment and in which the patient had clearly been released only to await death could be marked so that no follow-up is done. The call was just one more reminder of how much we had been through and how great my loss was.

There was a most unusual long distance phone call from a business acquaintance of Dan's, a man whom I had also known while working for the company. He had just heard about Dan's death and wanted to talk with me. He told me of the glories of the "other side" and said I should take comfort in knowing Dan was in such a wonderful place. He said he knew because he had seen it. A few years ago he had a very serious heart attack. There was a brief time when he saw a glimpse of the life beyond the grave. He had wanted to stay, but he could not. He was sent back. It was not yet time.

I was touched by his story and by his kindness in sharing it with me. Yes, I knew that if there were a place of glory, Dan would be there. I wasn't so sure I would ever qualify for entrance, and, oh, I missed him so!

I wished I could fall apart. Cry, scream, jump up and down, anything to release the feelings of tension and emptiness.

I studied the book my sister-in-law had given me, Rabbi Kushner's *When Bad Things Happen to Good People*. I agreed with most of his premise, but it provided me no solace. Only more confusion. I, too, could not love a God who would pick and choose among his followers. *"You can live. You must die."* Did He only set the world in motion and establish the natural laws? Are we now reaping the pain and the suffering from man's interference in those laws? Does God suffer, too, when His children suffer? I had felt that He was with us in the struggle, else we could not have faced each day. But now, where was He? It was as if He were hidden, even in church.

Even now, everyone says, "You are such a strong person." I wish I were half as strong as they seem to think I am. They ask how I feel, and I have to say, "Fine." No one wants to hear how I *really* feel. If I try to tell them, they interrupt with time-honored cliches. And so I keep quiet.

There is no anger. Who could I be angry at? There is sadness. Resentment. Especially when I see older couples together. Why are they still together? Some don't even like each other, while we, who loved so deeply and so well, are separated by death. Questions, always questions. Never any answers.

Perhaps I could give in to grief later. Now there was still work to do. I had called our attorney before leaving for Illinois to ask if there were any business I should take care of before I left. There wasn't. Dan and I had established our bank accounts in joint tenancy so sufficient funds were available. I ordered ten copies of the death certificate for I knew that a copy would have to be furnished to each insurance company and each financial institution in order to pay benefits and to transfer the assets into my name. Now it was time to take care of that paperwork.

I prepared an up-to-date list of all of our property and holdings and took it to our attorney. Our estate settlement would be simple, as all of the assets affected by Dan's death were in joint tenancy with right of survivorship. Though we had current wills, no probate procedures would be necessary. The attorney arranged for an appraisal of our home in order to establish the total value of Dan's estate for tax consideration and to establish a cost base as of the date the property became solely mine.

I called the Social Security office and wrote letters to the insurance companies and the Veterans Administration, then completed the forms which they furnished and returned them with a certified copy of Dan's death certificate so that benefits could be paid. I visited the Department of Motor Vehicles to clear title to the cars and to re-register them in my name. I also returned the Disabled Parking Permit. I had conferences with the attorney and visits with our broker. Each day brought more forms, more correspondence, more phone calls. I was thankful for my many years of business experience, especially in the field of insurance, so that the paperwork was not foreign to me.

When all this was completed, I prepared a new list of assets and made the decisions as to how to invest the insurance funds to protect my own future. This was followed by a new budget based upon my new needs as a single. I priced health insurance plans but fortunately I was eligible to continue coverage under the State Farm Group plan as the recipient of a portion of Dan's retirement pay.

And then there were the personal items.

I started sorting Dan's clothing. Handsome suits (one never worn) were sent to his brother. I shipped another box of good work suits and sports clothing to my nephew. Some went to the Salvation Army and still more to the Rescue Mission. Letting go of each item was like losing part of myself. I could not part with them all. His Navy uniform, tuxedo, a good wool suit and topcoat, I put into a garment bag and hung in the back of the closet.

I asked close friends to select an item of Dan's jewelry. One, a fellow Mason, wanted the boutonniere holder with the Masonic emblem on it; another, a set of cufflinks and tie tack. They were so pleased to share these items.

I cleaned out the drawer containing his lodge papers in order to return the manuals and code books to the lodge and found a cassette tape he had used in his memory work. I put it on the recorder and listened, paying no attention to the words, just that dear voice, and the tears flowed freely. Not only did I miss his touch, I missed the sound of his voice, the greeting when he returned home from work each night. Oh, how alone I felt!

I was not the only one to miss him. A friend stopped by and brought me a copy of the company newsletter containing Dan's memorial article and picture. I do not know who wrote this obituary, but I was touched by the last paragraph:

> Dan was a storehouse of knowledge and his coworkers regularly drew from that storehouse in the course of their daily work. All who worked closely with Dan and knew him well will miss him very much. We have lost one of this world's truly sincere individuals.

September 13, 1982

I do so hope this is the day I can finally get my act together—physically, emotionally and mentally. To shake this depression and accomplish something that would make Dan proud. While tea was brewing, I did our daily devotions in front of his picture. *Oh God, how I miss him!*

I will start a new diary, my own personal journal. Perhaps that will be a starting point to resume writing. I remember reading an article about Lady Bird Johnson in which she was quoted as saying that Lyndon had pushed, cajoled and loved her into doing things that were beyond her ability. Dan was the same way. He thought I could do anything, and with his faith, love and encouragement, I probably did accomplish much more than I would have been able to do otherwise. Probably even beyond the limits of my abilities. What will be the source of my strength and encouragement now?

October 11, 1982

Today I started on Dan's book. The title was easy: *Diary of Courage.* Throughout his two years of living with cancer, he was a positive inspiration to all who came into contact with him for his courage, his sense of humor, his continuing interest in their lives, his lack of complaint. These lives would continue to be touched by his wisdom, his tranquillity, his dignity as he lost his battle to live.

Could I find a small ray of that courage to take into my battle for a new and meaningful life? *To whom much is given, much will be required.* I had been given a special love. I would have to prove myself worthy.

My Prayer

My life must touch a million lives in some way ere I go
From this dear world of struggle to the land I do not know.
So this wish I always wish, the prayer I ever pray:
Let my life help the other lives it touches by the way!

Anonymous

Postscript

I WAS NOT TO BE ALLOWED my time of grieving. Mom had a severe heart attack in September and her condition worsened. On October 16 I flew back to Illinois to be with her, going straight from the airport to the hospital. The nurses greeted me with, "We're so glad you're here. She's been waiting for you." She rallied and a week later returned to her home. She would never be able to live alone again and my sister made arrangements to move in with her after I left.

During the two weeks I was there, I visited the cemetery. The Veterans Administration marker and the bronze vase had been installed. Dan's grave had been sodded and no longer had that new, raw look. Redwood chips were placed around the headstone and I put out a Thanksgiving wreath. It was a comfort to see how quickly his grave had blended in with those around him.

Upon my return to California I immediately visited Dan's mother. She had a virus and was not well, but the doctor had been to see her and she was resting comfortably. At 12:30 A.M., November 6, her doctor called. He thought she might have a blood clot in her right leg. What did I want him to do? I told him to call her son, and gave him Charles' phone number. Later when I visited her, the nurse had just given her a shot and she was sleeping. Still, I did our daily devotions and said a prayer. I hope she may have heard. At 3:40 A.M., Sunday, November 7, she quietly passed away in her sleep.

I made another trip to the mortuary. Charles and Sue arrived and we completed plans for a Memorial Service in Reno. Once again we went through the rites.

Every time I was on the verge of allowing grief to take over, some crisis arose and I had to pull myself together and get on with the business at hand.

I flew to Virginia and spent Christmas with Charles and Sue and their family.

Shortly after the first of the year, Mom's condition deteriorated so that my sister was no longer able to care for her. We went through the agony of getting her settled into a nursing home.

They say that the worst of the grief is over in three or four months, but during those months I was too busy coping with other crises to let myself grieve. Will I ever? I really don't know. I just keep on keeping on.

It is from the Psalmist that I seem to find my greatest comfort.

Whither shall I go from thy Spirit? or whither shall I flee from thy presence?

If I ascend up into heaven, thou *art* there: if I make my bed in hell, behold, thou *art there*.

If I take the wings of the morning, *and* dwell in the uttermost parts of the sea;

Even there shall thy hand lead me, and thy right hand shall hold me.

Psalms 139:7-10

Part 2—Sharing What We Learned

(Wounded Healers)

Living with the Patient

ANY LIFE-THREATENING ILLNESS involves not only the patient but his loved ones as well, and these loved ones, family and friends can do much to help the patient to cope and to maintain a meaningful quality of life.

During the early part of Dan's illness, I was overly protective of him, probably because of my past experience with cancer. My father had died from this disease at age fifty-six; his sister at age seventy-two. My maternal grandfather also died from cancer after living in constant pain for almost twenty years from the date of his first surgery. Then there were the hundreds of death and disability claims I had handled during my insurance career. These past but painful experiences affected both my confidence and my mood. I tried to keep a positive attitude, concentrating on the great strides made in cancer therapy in recent years. But the important lesson I learned was that it didn't make any difference how I felt, it was how *Dan* felt, *his* confidence, *his* acceptance of his condition, *his* fight for recovery that was important. I realized that I had to let him set the mood and set the pace. No one has the right to try to influence another human being in how to face a life or death struggle. Each person's life is his own. It was his inalienable right as the patient to determine how he would deal with his own destiny. I could best help him simply by following his lead and supporting him in his moods and in his decisions. In that manner, I could be his helpmate. I had no right to make demands upon his life. The choices were his. He was the one who decided not to have the hormone treatments. He elected surgery. When the surgery failed to stop the cancer, he chose the radiation treatments. He had no interest in chemotherapy. His choices. His decisions. I listened.

Let the Patient Set the Mood

Dan exhibited anger over his condition only briefly. It was during his last confinement at the acute care hospital after the ultimate prognosis had been given and while we were waiting for admission into the convalescent hospital. For a few days he wanted no visitors and he insisted that I stay constantly by his side. When I left for a brief respite, or even a cup of coffee, he became very agitated. A friend stopped by. He told me to make her go away. I realized it was not a personal anger directed at her, or at me. It was the anger of frustration, of being a prisoner of a condition and of a disease over which he had no control. The major cause of any distress is a feeling of loss of control. In no situation is this so true as in dealing with a medical problem.

Fear often entered my mind. Rarely did Dan show any evidence of special concern. During his recuperation period following the first hospital stay for the seizure-like episode, he occasionally expressed a fear of death and worry over finances. Our minister's regular visits and the books he brought for us to read seemed to remove any doubts from Dan's Christian beliefs. We kept our faith in God, in the doctors, in the treatments, in ourselves. I could and did reassure Dan as to our financial situation. When fear came up, we discussed its causes and found that it lessened with understanding. We seemed to have a balance. When my faith wavered, Dan's was strong. When his wavered, mine peaked. We both thought we had to be invincible because others depended upon us—his mother and mine. As a family of only two, we were also very dependent upon each other.

Though Dan shed no tears for himself, he was a most compassionate man who did cry for others' suffering. I believe it is important to allow anyone who is at a low ebb to complain and for others to listen to them, even agree with them, to let them know their feelings are valid. "Yes, it's the pits." After I lost him, I needed to have a good cry but no one would let me. How I longed for such release. At the time, I was not interested in the Pollyannas who told me how lucky I was. Since then, when friends face similar situations, I tell them, "Anytime you want to cry, or swear, or scream and want someone to listen, I'm here."

Our minister recently told the story of a worried father who started to scold his small daughter for being so late in coming home from school. "But," little Susan explained, "I was late because my friend Laura dropped her doll and it broke."

"I see," said the father, "you stayed to help her put her doll back together."

"No," replied Susan. "The doll was so broke we couldn't fix it. I stayed to help her cry."

As adults, when life is broke and can't be fixed, we also need someone to stay and help us cry.

When it became obvious to Dan that he was losing his fight, he confronted it openly and honestly, acknowledging and accepting his fate. If he had preferred living with illusions, then I would have had to share those with him, though personally, I do not believe in the current popular theory that one can get well simply by positive thinking. It is just that each individual has his/her own way of dealing with reality. This applies to many aspects of life, not just illness. It is up to family and friends to follow the lead of the patient.

While Dan's moods were usually positive and his emotions well-controlled, I had more difficulty with my own. He was so optimistic that his course of treatment would cure him. During this time, I kept my doubts and fears to myself. I hope that I was able to disguise the intense guilt I felt at not being able to care for him at home during the last few weeks of his life. I was not trained in patient care. I could not lift him or turn him by myself. I did not know how to treat bedsores. He constantly needed changes in medication for pain relief. His condition required care far beyond my ability to handle at home without 24-hour assistance. Even if such assistance had been available, we both had fears that the help might not be reliable, that it might not show up as scheduled, or would not have sufficient skill to meet all his needs. He had doubts about home care. So did I, but that didn't make me feel any less inadequate. We each have different strengths and different weaknesses. As a result, the support we can give our loved ones takes different forms. We cannot be all things to our loved ones, much as we would want. We must each do our personal best and turn a deaf ear to those who criticize. I just had to forgive myself for the things I couldn't do. And while there were limits to the physical care I could provide, there was no limit to the emotional support I could give. I kept this thought uppermost in my mind.

Dan seemed at peace after he realized he would be able to stay at the convalescent hospital, would not be moved again, and would get good care. He had his plateaus when his condition would be maintained for several days, a time when he seemed no weaker, perhaps even stronger. Then there would be a further decline—the loss of ability to keep oral medicine down, adjustment to a new medication, difficulty with swallowing and maintaining food. New medicines would be tried; his condition would stabilize and he would be fairly comfortable for a few days. Then that medication no longer quelled the pain and there would be further deterioration in his condition.

Those plateaus were the most difficult for me to deal with. Sometimes I could almost envision his getting well, though I knew that was not possible. Then the downturns. It was like a roller coaster. But the patient was on the same roller coaster, so we rode it together.

I believe that some of Dan's strength was born in his genes. He reminded me of his father who, when struck with a second major heart attack and confined for six weeks in a hospital, read his Bible in Greek, Latin and English. I also believe that we all have that strength within us. We just have to learn how to reach it and the methods are as diverse as we are. We all need someone to listen to our problems, and sometimes that is all we need to find our strength—just someone to listen as we express our concerns aloud.

Listen

When I ask you to listen to me
And you start giving advice
You have not done when I asked.

When I ask you to listen to me
And you begin to tell me why I shouldn't feel the way I do
You are trampling on my feelings.

Listen!
All I asked was that you listen.
Not talk, or advise—just listen.

Advice is cheap.
Newspapers, magazines and books are filled with advice.
I can search it out for myself.

I'm not helpless.
Suffering, discouraged, faltering.
But not helpless.

I need you to listen;
To accept the fact that I do feel as I feel.
If you will just listen, I can sort things out in my own mind
And find the answers.
And I don't need your advice.

From *First Christian Church Courier*.

Let the Patient Set the Pace

Early on, Dan showed me that he would yield no quarter to his cancer. We kept busy. We lived our normal lives and ignored the threat of his illness as much as possible. When Dan started his series of radiation treatments, I again became overly-protective as I had at the time of the first diagnosis. I knew the radiation was killing healthy cells along with the diseased and that weakness would result. I was afraid of his twisting, falling, lifting, causing broken bones, but life had no meaning or purpose to him unless he could do some of the things he enjoyed. He worked every day until he became too weak to make it to the office. One of his colleagues told me he didn't see how Dan got up from the chair behind his desk at times, but he did. When he had to give up his golf, he continued to walk daily. He attended church and lodge and the camera club meetings in pain because he enjoyed these activities. They were an important part of his life and he intended to live fully as long as strength would allow. I could have spoiled his days if I had insisted that he take it easy. So when he wanted to go out to dinner, we went and had a good time. Whatever he felt he could do, we did.

Family and Friends

I overheard a cancer patient say, "First you lose your friends, then you lose your hair."

When we first learned of the nature of Dan's illness, we kept the news to ourselves, except for immediate family and a few intimate friends. We were aware that it is a subject many people simply cannot deal with. Also, we were so confident of Dan's recovery that we wanted no stigma attached to us either from a social or from an economic standpoint. During this time, the letters and phone calls which we received from our loved ones were a constant source of our strength and well-being.

It was only when Dan's condition reached the point that he could no longer work that his illness became generally known. From that time on, the support of our minister and our church, family, and friends became an even more important part of our strength and our courage. His lodge brothers, colleagues from work, fraternity brothers and friends from college days, relationships we had built through the years were crucial to our emotional health.

We did, of course, lose some of those who just couldn't handle cancer, death or dying—even Dan's mother for a time. Many people insulate themselves and distance themselves from trouble. These people do not mean to be thoughtless or neglectful; it is just that they have not yet dealt with their own mortality and until they do, they will continue to deprive themselves of the rewards of sharing love and compassion with those who have.

But a visit with Dan was not the usual sickroom visit. There was no talk of either getting well or dying from him. He was only interested in his visitors, their work and their activities, the outside world. His was not a room of sorrow but of faith. He would talk and laugh with them and each visitor went away uplifted, though beyond the closed door there were tears in their eyes as they talked with me and I comforted them. I did not discourage these visits, even though near the end they had to be of short duration. He was the one to indicate if he was tired or ready to rest. He salvaged the maximum pleasure possible from his last days by keeping his spirits upbeat. I could certainly do no less.

When I left his room at night, however, I could not face dinner alone and until my sister arrived, friends and neighbors frequently shared their meals with me.

Dan and I were private people, members of a generation who are not attuned to use of agencies or community resources or even aware of most of them. We were raised in a time and in an environment in which each family took care of its own and though we were only two, we were still a family. Social workers, government or private agencies were simply not a part of our life or even a part of our lexicon. We felt that we should get our medical information and treatment from our doctors, that they are the experts, and that love and support should come from friends and associations we had established through the years.

But just as cancers are all different, so are people's reactions to cancer equally different. Some people want to know all about their illness and take an active role in their treatment. Others, such as noted columnist Guy Wright, express a different view. He wrote, concerning his own cancer, "Quite early I decided I couldn't become an instant expert on cancer. I would only burn up a lot of energy trying, energy needed for healing." [*San Francisco Examiner*, July 21, 1985.]

One day I brought home a book on cancer entitled *Getting Well Again*. Dan would not read it. At the time, he knew he was losing his fight and he didn't want to read someone else's thoughts on winning theirs.

Although the survival rates for certain types of cancers have improved through the years, the chances of survival are still grim— approximately 50 per cent will die within five years. If you are exposed only to positive and successful experiences, you feel a personal sense of failure because you are not winning, life is not turning out that way for you in spite of all your struggle. I'm sure that he would have been interested in Rabbi Harold Kushner's book *When Bad Things Happen to Good People*, but we didn't know about this valuable book then.

Some people view death as the end of all. We believe that death is not the closing of the book, but simply the ending of one chapter and the beginning of another. Our experience developed within us a philosophy that we should live each day as if we would live forever *and* as if we would die tomorrow and do it simultaneously.

Other Sources of Support

While we sought and received support from existing contacts, each patient must seek his own source of faith and courage and each family must adapt to the patient's decision. There is no one all-inclusive answer. The important goal is to find that source which best suits the needs of the individual patient and his/her family.

1. The American Cancer Society
   This organization has several programs on cancer. *CanSurmount* is a short-term visitor program for patients, and the families of patients, with many types of cancer, done on a one-to-one basis.

   Group programs such as *I Can Cope* provide information on cancer therapy, treatment, side effects, nutrition, resource availability and other topics of interest to cancer patients and their families.

   They also have other programs for patients coping with

specific types of cancer such as *Reach to Recovery* for breast cancer, *Laryngectomy Rehabilitation Program* and *Ostomy Rehabilitation Program*.

2. Council on Aging
    While dealing mostly with senior citizens, the Council on Aging has valuable information on various services available in the community.

3. Hospital Chaplaincy Program
    In our community, this program provides trained volunteers to visit patients and listen to their concerns.

4. Home Hospice
    Our local hospice has caregiver volunteers, a referral service and also a bereavement program.

5. Church, Lodge, Other Organizations
    Our church has a "Caring Corps" to visit shut-ins. Dan's lodge had available for loan various items of equipment, such as commodes and walkers.

6. Library
    Local libraries are a good source to determine what agencies and groups are active in the community. They also have many books on illnesses such as cancer, hence my reason for writing this book: To share experiences with other patients and families.

7. Private Counseling
    There are many licensed marriage and family counselors and social workers who specialize in therapy for patients and families.

Helpful Hints

When illness strikes, we become aware of the lack of facilities in our homes, items that should be and are now becoming more standard in homebuilding. Even before a life-threatening situation arises, people fall and break bones, necessitating the use of crutches or walkers. Every house should be adapted to include guard rails beside all steps, grab bars in bathrooms and showers, no-slip floors in showers and tubs, higher toilet seats. We need to eliminate throw rugs, aptly named.

As soon as Dan's mobility was limited, I secured a form from the Department of Motor Vehicles which his doctor completed entitling us to a disabled parking permit.

We found that a fabric or vinyl pouch, such as those fastened onto bicycle handlebars are easily attached to walkers, enabling the patient to carry tissues, a cordless phone, and other necessities around with him. A plastic glass with lock-type cover can be used to carry beverages. Orthopedic supply companies have all kinds of adaptive equipment for walking, feeding, bathing and self-care. Insurance may help pay for these with a doctor's prescription.

Pillows made out of egg-crate mattresses make sitting more comfortable; they also elevate the seat of the chair, making it easier to rise from. The new patient kits from the hospital are equally helpful at home with their plastic glasses, urinals, bedpans, and wash trays.

I cut a plastic garbage bag along one side to make a cover for the mattress. A plastic mat by the side of the bed saved the carpet from many an accident. Waterproof Chux will protect the bedding, and disposable adult diapers such as Depends can make the patient feel more secure about getting up to walk and going out in public; both are available from hospital supply stores and many pharmacies.

Jogging suits make warm and comfortable clothing that is easy to get into, and they are equally appropriate indoors and outside. For patients with catheters, the pants must be large enough to allow the bag to be passed down through the pants leg. Women can more easily dress themselves in housecoats and dresses that fasten in the front. Velcro tennis shoes can be put on with only one hand and are safer for walking than leather-soled shoes or slippers, also aptly named.

Pill-holders, those containers which provide space for a week's supply of medication, help to avoid errors and omissions.

A cordless phone gives the patient security when left alone. Many hospitals offer a service, such as Lifeline, where they rent an alarm about the size of a watch to be worn on the wrist or around the neck. If the subscriber needs assistance, the alarm button is pushed. The hospital will then call the subscriber. If there is no answer, they will then call a friend or family member to check on the patient. If there is still no response, an ambulance is dispatched. For many people living alone, this is truly a "lifeline."

Maintaining a routine as near to normal as possible is important to keep the patient from feeling like an invalid. Even after Dan was unable to work, I helped him to shave, bathe and dress every morning. When we went to his doctors' appointments, he made a selection from his wardrobe of caps and hats to cover up his sparse hair while it was growing out from the radiation therapy. His barber, a friend of long-standing, came to the hospital and also out to the house to keep his hair in trim. Good grooming was a great ego-builder!

Since we spent many hours there, it was helpful to both Dan and me to make the room at the convalescent hospital homey.

I got permission to hang pictures on the walls and to put up a clock with numbers large enough for him to read from his bed. There were always flowers on his bedside table and a transistor radio, never used. We had our Bible, the *Daily* Word and the *Upper* Room for our daily devotions. A basket held cards and letters which arrived every day. He had his chair from home and a family afghan. Though he wore only gowns in the hospital, he wore his own robe when he was lifted from bed for meals. One jogging suit hung in the closet—just to be there.

I regret that we did not have a register for our visitors to sign. There were so many of them. Some came daily. It would be comforting to have such a record.

Personal Medical Records

EARLY ON WE WISHED that we had maintained our own personal medical records. When Dan first told me of the possibility of prostate cancer, I remembered the tests he'd had during the early years of our marriage, when we were still hoping to have a family. Those tests revealed a low sperm count. His doctor was unconcerned, however, as "there were still enough to do the job." Any deficiency was attributed to the stress in his work. During the recent past, when there were occasions of impotency, his doctor had also blamed stress at work and the advancing years. Early fifties? Could this have started long ago, I wondered. Did his doctor simply miss it, or not examine him or his records sufficiently to make a diagnosis?

When he gave evidence of an allergic reaction, we also felt the clues to the problem were in his files. At one time he had been given a series of shots and he was warned not to have any more of the substance administered. We both had forgotten what the particular substance was. We thought they had been iron shots, but we were unable to verify this. We talked with his former doctor in the Bay Area who had sent a summary of his records to the doctor in Santa Rosa. Neither of them acknowledged any such information. We wondered how complete the records were that were transferred, and how thoroughly they had been studied by his new physician.

At the time, the patient did not have access to the information in his medical records. California Health & Safety Code, Sections 25250-25258, now give California residents the right to read their records within five working days by making written request and paying reasonable clerical costs and to get copies within fifteen days of a written request. One local hospital charges a fee of $10.00 plus $.25 per page after the first six pages. Several other states have similar legislation. A Uniform Health-Care Information Act has been developed and started through the state legislative process in 1987. It is hoped that eventually there will be some uniformity in accessing records for all patients. In the interim, however, you can write to The American Medical Record Association, 875 N. Michigan Ave., Suite 1850, Chicago, IL 60611 for information on regulations in your state.

Public Law 93-579, the Privacy Act of 1974, governs the rights of patients to access records of treatment in federal medical care facilities such as Veterans Administration hospitals.

The physician may still be allowed to determine which patients may see their records and may limit access if the release of records directly to the patient would be medically unwise. Some doctors believe seeing the full records would frighten the patient, but others, like Boston University's George Annas, author of *The Rights of Hospital Patients*, an American Civil Liberties Union guide, believe that seeing your records "can be a powerful means of health education," can be useful for "checking the accuracy of family and personal histories," and for giving more informed consent to future treatment. [*San Francisco Chronicle*, April 24, 1985. Victor Cohn.]

Still, such legislation does not solve all the problems. Doctors retire. We move. Records are lost or incomplete, sometimes inaccurate, or even destroyed after a period of time. At the time of my last major surgery, the anesthesiologist told me there had been problems with the medication and anesthesia administered (I knew I had become violently ill) and that these medicines should not be used on me in the future. I did not record the information (I was barely conscious at the time) and forgot about it until recently, when I was to undergo some minor surgery and I remembered the admonition. When I contacted the surgeon, he said he found no notation about the anesthetic in his records but that this information would normally be shown on the surgical records at the hospital. I then contacted the hospital, gave the date of the surgery, and was informed that their records for that year had been destroyed. Fortunately, medicines have been improved; however, I still wish I knew the names of those which had proved so troublesome.

Though patients have a legal right to the essential information in their records in a doctor's office or hospital, it is rare that there is an opportunity to review those records for completeness, accuracy or timeliness. Frequently, potentially dangerous and costly diagnostic x-rays and tests are repeated by a new doctor rather than waiting for the records from another source, though it would be in the patient's best interests and far safer to apply pressure to get these test results and records.

A procedure may also be repeated because the doctor does not check to see if it has already been done. When Dan was first admitted to the hospital, the neurologist ordered a second CAT-scan when he was unable to make a diagnosis from the first. This duplication was necessary. However, an x-ray imaging of his entire body was done on February 1 and only five days later his physician ordered x-rays of the femurs to determine whether or not to start physical therapy. This seems to me now [I did not know about it at the time] to have been useless and unnecessary.

Stanford University's Dr. Eugene Robin, author of *Medical Care Can Be Dangerous to Your Health*, states that during the past ten years, doctors have become increasingly aware of the dangers of x-rays, even the low-dose diagnostic x-rays, due to the cumulative buildup in one's system. He advises that one should keep some sort of record of x-rays and other diagnostic procedures so that when the doctor orders another, the patient can say, "Wait a minute. I had such and such done on (date). Is this really necessary?"

In this age of specialization we deal with many doctors who know very little about us and who would benefit from information in another doctor's file. Each such specialist does not have our complete records, but instead, only those he has prepared concerning the specific problem he is treating. Yet we are not a collection of fragmented, unrelated parts that can be treated individually, as a mechanic might treat a car. We are whole persons and it is our whole person that must be treated.

Each doctor has a tendency to start from here and now, ignoring the past, yet there must be a relationship between past health history and current ailments. We humans, at least mentally and emotionally, are the sum total of our past experiences. Why are we not physically the result of past illnesses and injuries? There is a universal exposure to causative agents, but at what point is the body no longer able to resist?

New studies recognize the importance of genetics as a factor in disease, its prevention and treatment. A recent article on the immune system reported that memory cells remember the various germs that have attacked in the past and these cells trigger the immune system if the same germ attacks again. But when and why does the immune system fail or break down? Surely part of the answer lies in the amount of work it has already been called upon to do. This information is in our personal medical history, just as the genetic factor is revealed in our family medical history.

In reviewing our records in preparation for writing this book, I felt that I, as a layman, could distinguish a pattern relating to Dan's illness, yet none of the doctors who treated him ever seemed to give any thought to his past medical history.

Of equal concern to the patient is the question of just how thoroughly the doctor studies the medical records which do exist. In insurance, we would never see a customer or attempt to answer his inquiry without carefully reviewing his file to be certain we knew all details. Is this done in medicine?

My sister suffered from osteoporosis, a battle which resulted in eight surgical procedures within five years. I was with her during her surgery in March 1986. As this was a teaching hospital, students, nurses, residents and aides frequently interrupted her rest to ask questions about her condition and her past medical history, the answers to which were in her file. I'm sure my sister's lengthy medical history and the progression of her disease were an important learning experience; however, I feel some discretion should be used and consideration should be given to how much this disturbs the patient. A year later, she consulted her orthopedic surgeon for her broken hip. He explained that he would put a pin in it, but she reminded him that he had tried inserting a pin into her broken leg, a break which had not healed in more than eighteen months, and that the pin didn't work.

"Oh yes," he replied. "That's right." Then he went on to explain about putting in a new socket. What would have happened if my sister had not reminded him of the previous experience?

Though the medical record is the physical property of the health care practitioner or facility who compiles it, they own only the pieces of paper upon which the record is written—the information is the patient's. What do these records contain? Information about the patient, information provided by the patient to a physician who is being paid by the patient, and x-ray films and the results of diagnostic tests for which the patient has also paid. This information is vital to the patient if he is to be knowledgeable about his own health care and should be readily accessible to him. In the military, medical records are given to patients to take with them as they are transferred from place to place. Why not the same procedure in private life?

Blue Cross and Blue Shield of Maryland have been working on a project through which their subscribers would receive membership cards that can contain the equivalent of eight hundred pages of information on their medical history, including x-rays and electrocardiograms. These cards would be wallet-sized so they could be carried on the insured's person; however, the information on the cards could be read only by means of personal computer and laser optics technology and therefore would not be readily available to the patient himself.

We realized that personal medical records are valuable for all of the following reasons:

1. to avoid duplication of costly and potentially hazardous x-rays and diagnostic procedures;
2. to more intelligently discuss our condition and treatment with our doctors;
3. because of the continued research and knowledge of the importance of genetic predisposition in disease development;
4. because it is important to know how the immune system has performed in the past;
5. and because doctor and hospital records may be lost, incomplete, inaccurate, or inaccessible.

We established a record, as best we could, from memory, from reviewing income tax returns on which we had claimed medical expense deductions and from conversations with our families. We then started keeping more complete current information. Ideally, such records should be started at birth, kept up-to-date and then given to each child as they leave home.

Personal medical records may be in any format, perhaps a loose-leaf notebook with a section for each member of the family, but should include all of the following:

- Patient's name
- Date of visit
- Problem, symptoms, or complaint
- Doctor's name, address and phone number
- Diagnosis and treatment
- Medication prescribed, including name, dosage, potency, period of time to be taken, side effects
- Reaction to medication
- Any other treatment or tests, such as x-rays
- Amount paid
- Insurance company, name and address
- Amount paid by insurance
- Net expense (total less insurance)

Obviously, such records would be helpful in completing insurance claim forms and income tax returns. Dental care should be included since x-rays are a part of a dental checkup and it would be well to also include eye examinations.

The People's Medical Society has a printed form for such records, though they do not include any space for costs and reimbursements. Their forms are available by writing to them at 462 Walnut St., Allentown, PA 18102. Current cost (1989) is $4.00.

I have also included copies of some forms which I prepared.

The entries into the medical record should be made promptly after each doctor's visit, while the information is still fresh in your mind. Don't try to reconstruct it later.

We found our records, as incomplete as they were, were helpful to us in preparing for the next visit with each doctor. After reviewing them, we prepared a list of specific questions we wanted answered and wrote down their answers. This made us feel more in control.

Name _____

Date of Birth _____ Place of Birth _____

Insurance Company _____ Policy No. or Identification _____

Social Security No. _____

Date	Doctor or Hospital / Name, Address, Phone	Complaint/symptoms	Diagnosis/Treatment	Cost	Insurance Paid	Net

Name _____

Drugs & Medications (including over-the-counter, vitimins & minerals)

Date	Name of Medication	Doctor	Pharmacy	Dosage & Period Taken	Side Effects/Reactions	Cost	Ins. Paid	Net

X-Rays / Diagnostic Tests

Name _____

Date	Name of Lab and/or Doctor	Test Performed	Results	Cost	Ins. Paid	Net

Doctor/Patient Relationships

"Dr. J.W. Woodard
Physician and Surgeon

Ladies and gentlemen—one and all,
  If you get sick give me a call
And I will come with main and might
  Either by day or a dark night.

I will come with a free will—
  (Hoping you will not murmur at your bill;)
I pledge my word I will not rue,
  If you will pay up when it's due."

This advertisement of my great-great-great-uncle appeared in the Clinton, Illinois *Central Transcript* of October 20, 1864. To earn his living, he also ran a small farm. Earlier, my great-great-great-grandfather, Dr. Jesse McPherson, had been a doctor, county coroner and Methodist preacher in order to support his family.

Samuel Sanes, M.D. wrote in his book *A Physician Faces Cancer in Himself* that the doctor's charge used to be "to cure when possible, relieve when indicated, comfort and console always." Now, with modern technology, "he looks at patients in terms of overcoming disease in as rapid a time as possible, or holding it in check over the long term. He is liable to think less about relief and almost not at all about comfort and consolation. With the waxing of the science of medicine, the art of medicine has waned."

During the past eleven years I have been intimately exposed to doctors and the modern health-care delivery system, beginning with my mother-in-law's stroke in April 1978, followed by Dan's diagnosis of cancer in July 1980, my sister's battle with osteoporosis which ended with her death in June 1988, and my mother's long-term heart disease which took her life in May 1989. I have spent many hours in doctors' offices, hospitals and clinics, observing, listening, learning. I have learned that of all the changes which have occurred in recent years, none so personally touches our lives as the changes in the doctor/patient relationship.

I was born on a farm in Illinois; Dan, in a small town in Nevada.

Until we each left home after high school, we had been cared for by the doctors who had helped to bring us into the world. During our years in the San Francisco Bay Area we were treated by physicians who were of the old school, who were concerned with us both as individuals and as a family. Three years after our move to Santa Rosa, I returned to the Bay Area for surgery to be performed by the same doctor who had operated on me previously. We decided, however, we should have a family doctor closer to where we lived.

We found our new family physician by accident, a referral by the local medical society as the only physician who made house calls when I was down, literally, with a back spasm. We had only brief contacts with him until Dan went for a complete physical in 1975. Between 1975 and 1980 we had rarely seen him. When the life-threatening condition arose, we had not had sufficient experience with this doctor to know if he would meet our needs. Then we immediately became involved in the physician referral service, so that by the time it was evident he could not provide the warmth of caring and support we needed, Dan's illness had reached the point that no useful purpose would be served by making a change. It was too late.

The Referral Service

"You are scared and sick and going to all these doctors, but none of them is talking to each other," said a fellow cancer patient.

From our background of small towns and family doctors, we were thrust headlong into the world of modern medicine, into an arena of specialists.

The first specialist we were referred to was the urologist. Dan saw him only twice; I met him once, before the surgery. He was curt to the point of seeming unfriendly. He offered no word of sympathy, no suggestions for counseling, no advice. But we thought that since he had the confidence of our family doctor, he must be good at his specialty. His skill was our primary concern. After all, we expected the surgery to be successful; therefore we would see little of him. Dan was only to be his patient temporarily.

When Dan's pain returned, he visited his family physician, then returned to the urologist who remained uncommunicative and who gave him an additional referral to a radiologist. This specialist became a friend. He took time to talk with us both, to explain the treatments, the side effects and to answer our questions. Since we saw him daily over a period of time, he became the first doctor we called in an emergency, even though we should have called the family physician and ultimately did.

When Dan was first admitted to the emergency care unit at the hospital in a seizure-like state, I tried to explain to the doctor on duty about his cancer, that his bones had been decimated by the cancer and the radiation, and that the uncontrolled jerking movements caused him excruciating pain. Instead of listening to me, he ordered me from the room. It was not until our personal physician arrived that any consideration was given to Dan's condition. His relief was delayed because of lack of knowledge and the fact that the doctor would not accept my explanation. Later in the day, our own doctor left the hospital and returned to his office without giving me any information. If only he had come to me and said, "I don't know what's causing this . . . I don't know what has happened . . . I've ordered a series of tests to determine, diagnose . . ." He simply left. It was the radiologist who called in the neurologist for us. This specialist understood my need to know and allowed me to accompany Dan for some of his tests. He also talked with us freely, even though his participation in Dan's care was limited.

There are problems, however, associated with the referral service. Dealing with a series of specialists can be as puzzling, foreign and frustrating as the disease itself. We felt that no single doctor understood Dan's overall condition—that each was concerned only with his own specialty. None of them really knew Dan. They didn't know he would mention pain only if it was intolerable. Did his lack of complaint adversely affect his care? If radiation had started immediately when his pain returned instead of nine months later, would it have been more successful?

Though the doctors attempted to keep each other informed, there were communication gaps, for example, repetition of tests. There were also some problems with coordination of medications.

We were confused as to who we should call when emergencies arose. The public is frequently criticized for excessive use of emergency facilities; however, some of this could be the result of the "specialist system." We simply don't know who to call, or the doctor we would normally rely on is not available.

Communication

Specialization is not the only problem. Other factors affect our efforts to establish good rapport with a physician, and while it is not reasonable to expect that every doctor we meet will serve our emotional needs, or be easy to talk with, especially as we are referred from specialist to specialist, it is essential that we find a primary care physician (family doctor) whose personality suits our needs.

A major cause of conflicts between doctor and patient is lack of communication. There is an old clinical adage that says "If you let the person tell you what's wrong, they will." The American Society of Internal Medicine reported that "Doctors of internal medicine—internists—have found that over 70 per cent of correct diagnoses are made through dialogue with the patient." [*The Press Democrat.* June 1, 1986.]

We older patients grew up in a time when the doctor was a father figure and we were in awe of them, their training and their profession. We are still somewhat intimidated by them, respectful of them and we treat them with dignity; yet studies show doctors spend less time with older patients than with younger. Obviously, we have to get their attention.

Usually, we do not visit a doctor unless there is something wrong with us and we are already worried and not a little frightened. Since we are vulnerable at this particular time, we want the doctor to be larger than life, superior. Though being in control is one of the primary motives in behavior, in our concern we give up that control, temporarily at least, turning it over to them, hoping they can make everything all right.

Our awe is slowly replaced by doubts and disappointments as we realize the limits of the doctor's knowledge and abilities and the meaning of those limitations to us in our life and death situations. Modern medical technology has been oversold. This is acknowledged even by the experts.

Victor C. Strasburger, a physician who practices pediatrics in southwestern Connecticut writes that "Part of the problem is that medicine has not come nearly as far as most people believe . . . Being treated in this new, modern age is no guarantee of a successful outcome" and that "if doctors took the time to carefully explain the risks and benefits of treatment, patients' expectations might not be sky-high. Everything in medicine has its risks . . . and doctors know this. They simply don't always take the time to communicate it to their patients." [*San Francisco Chronicle-Examiner*. April 6, 1986.]

We were never advised of possible side effects of any medication, yet Dan did suffer from allergic reactions. He became constipated, and not until later did we learn that constipation is a common reaction to the use of codeine. Butazolidin was one of the drugs prescribed for Dan; yet *Parade* [June 16, 1985] reported that this drug was banned in Sweden, Norway, Israel and several other countries as extremely dangerous. The new drug mentioned by his urologist came to our attention much too late to be of help. Should this have been made known to us sooner? In time to be of help?

I could not convince the doctors that Dan should have food supplements to help to restore his body, yet I have heard from other physicians on radio and television that no diet of 1,200 calories or less provides sufficient vitamins or minerals and that supplements are needed. Doctors seem to know so little about nutrition, vitamins, minerals, fuel for the body they are trying to heal.

And our doubts turn to fears as we learn how technology may be used not to alleviate suffering but to prolong it. We read of patients hooked up to life-support systems against their will and against the will of their family. We read of the malpractice suits and the reports of estimates that approximately 15 per cent of physicians are incompetent or impaired.

We are constantly sifting through conflicting information. An article on the annual physical [*Parade*, December 28, 1986.] stated that medical experts have reexamined the evidence and concluded that healthy people without symptoms do not need a total health screening every year and don't routinely need certain procedures, among them the rectal exam. Yet cancer is called the silent killer because it does not show symptoms and we are advised to pursue early detection. Prostate cancer is the third leading cause of cancer death in men, and once cancer spreads beyond the prostate gland, 80 per cent of the patients die within a decade. Dr. John K. Lattimer, chairman emeritus of the urology department of Columbia University was quoted as saying that "those whose cancer has grown large enough to explode to other parts of the body will die a death that might have been prevented." [*Parade*, July 22, 1984. "The Operation That Men Fear Most," by Randi Londer.]

Would a more thorough exam have revealed Dan's cancer in time to have saved his life?

Dorothea Lynch in her book, *Exploding Into Life*, wrote: "No one at the outpatient clinic tells me that radiation burns. No one tells me the steroids will make me a space-cadet, wheeling around like a pinwheel, unable to pull a word from my head, to think a coherent thought."

Dr. Dean Edell was quoted as saying, "People have a right to know what we know. They've been getting the run-around for too long." [*San Francisco Chronicle*. November 19, 1986.]

But lines of communication run both ways. Doctors must realize that sometimes the patient shuts them off. When he gives us information we're not prepared to deal with, or he uses a medical term with which we are not familiar, we tune him out trying to cope with our fears or to figure out the meaning. They must give us time to accept something that may come as a shock, such as a diagnosis of cancer. They should use words we understand. It is not necessary to say "metastasis." They can explain that the cancer has spread. Remember, we the patients hire the doctor to perform a service, and part of that service is to provide useful information that makes sense to us.

Other Concerns

Dr. Charles V. Ford, former chief of psychiatry at Wadsworth Veterans Administration Hospital in Los Angeles has stated that we are becoming a nation of hypochondriacs with our preoccupation with health.[Charles V. Ford *San Francisco Chronicle-Examiner*, October 12, 1986.] But it is only because we have lost some of our faith in the medical care delivery system.

Besieged as we are, both doctor and patient, by outside intervention from government in the form of Medicare and Medicaid, insurance companies, employers and the law, it is more important than ever before for doctor and patient to work together if we are to salvage and retain quality in our medical care. Decisions that were previously private, between doctor and patient, now seem to be affairs of the public, and we both have the added stress of loss of control over our own destiny. A recent survey revealed almost one-half of the nation's doctors feel pressure to release Medicare patients before they're ready. The doctors also have to cope with hospital review committees looking over their shoulders. Doctors and patients are caught in this web of specialization, modern technology and cost containment. This is not likely to change.

What Can We Do?

We must find a personal physician, internist or family practitioner, with whom we can communicate and in whom we have confidence. This physician will be our first line of defense in our care and must be willing, if necessary, to coordinate our treatment with consultants with whom we are not always comfortable, who will see us only for their own specialty. Our primary care physician must be one who knows us, knows our family and looks at us as whole persons, not collections of interchangeable parts. This physician's knowledge of our health, our family history and our personalities can be more valuable than a lot of expensive tests. The time and energy we spend finding such a physician could very well save a life and certainly salvage our peace of mind. The search must be done when we're well—not when ill and in need of treatment.

We can start by collecting the names of physicians in our area. A call to the local medical society will give referrals. We can contact a teaching hospital or nearby medical school and ask for the names of primary care physicians who take private patients. Local hospitals can provide lists of internists and family practitioners on their staff. We can talk with pharmacists and nurses we know. They deal regularly with local physicians. Our friends and relatives are another source, and when we move to a new location, our present physician may be able to recommend someone for us to contact.

Before making an appointment, we can check to see whether the physician is board-certified in internal medicine or family practice by checking the *Directory of Medical Specialists* in the public library. The *American Medical Directory*, also available at the library, lists all licensed physicians, some of whom aren't board-certified. Also, with a call to the physician's office, we can find out hospital affiliations, whether or not he makes house calls and whether or not he is a member of a group practice. A group practice ensures that another physician will be available on our physician's day off; otherwise, we need to determine who covers for him when he is not available.

We can schedule a first visit simply to have blood pressure

checked or talk with the doctor. Though one hates to go to a doctor unless it is absolutely necessary, we must see the physician often enough to determine if our needs will be met. Does she really listen to us when we talk? Is he impatient with our questions? Are we comfortable with her ? Does his office and staff provide a pleasant and caring environment? Find out whatever is important. If she does not meet our requirements, then we must continue our search until we find a doctor who does.

We must let our doctor know what we expect, keeping in mind he is only human. Do we want to know all we can about any illness or problem, or do we wish to defer to her judgment? Do we want to be kept alive by any available means, or is there some limit we would want to establish to our treatment? We need to know if the doctor will accede to our wishes on these very important matters. We would be on a collision course if he were to pursue aggressive treatment against the wishes of the patient and the family.

Before we make any visit to any doctor, we should prepare a list of specific questions we want answered. A review of our personal medical records (discussed in a previous chapter) will help us to compile this list and assemble any other information our doctor should have concerning our family health and past treatment. With this information at hand, we can more intelligently discuss our current problems.

Canadian physician Sir William Osler wrote more than a half century ago that "a patient with a written list of symptoms" suffers "neurasthenia" or mental upset, and as recently as 1969 a British medical text said note-writing is "almost a sure sign of psychoneurosis." [*San Francisco Chronicle*. December 4, 1986. "Body Talk," by Victor Cohn.] Nevertheless, we found, and it is now generally well-accepted, that to get the information one needs from his doctor, one should arrive at the office with a well-prepared list of symptoms and questions and leave space for answers to be recorded on the spot. Though the answers were not always forthcoming—we should have insisted—I'm sure we did get more information than we would have received if not prepared.

A suggested list of questions include:

- What's the diagnosis? Ask for a translation, if needed.
- What is this test you're ordering?
- Why is it necessary?

- Is it dangerous?
- What do the test results mean?
- What are the available treatments? Choices?
- What are the risks and the benefits?
- What will happen if I do nothing?

When the doctor gives us a prescription, we should tell him exactly what other medicines, vitamins or minerals we are taking and whether or not we drink alcohol. Some medicines should be taken before meals, some with meals, some after meals, some never with milk or dairy products.

We need to ask:

- What is the name of the medication?
- What is it supposed to do?
- How do I take it and for how long?
- What foods, drinks, other medicines or activities should I avoid while taking this medicine?
- What are the side effects? What should I do if they occur?
- Is there any written information available about this medication?

It is also well to discuss the medication with your pharmacist at the time you have the prescription filled and always read the printed information enclosed with the medicine. We found the Public Affairs Pamphlets, No. 570, *Know Your Medication* and No. 515, *Drugs—Use, Misuse, Abuse Guidance for Families,* most helpful. For information, write to Public Affairs Pamphlets, 381 Park Ave. South, New York 10016.

In spite of our lists of questions, however, we patients must still rely on the doctor to volunteer to us the information we need for informed consent for our treatment and to ensure the treatment's chances for success. In many instances, we will simply not be sufficiently knowledgeable to know the pertinent questions to ask.

It is helpful not to go to the doctor alone, for two sets of ears are better than one, and a family member or friend can be remote enough from the situation to better remember or understand what the doctor says. Many doctors, however, will discourage any intrusion into their strictly doctor/patient relationship. I encountered doctors who appeared irritated when I asked a question Dan had not brought up, as if it were none of my business. But it is important to make sure we get all the information that concerns us.

"Greater emphasis should be placed on the doctor's responsibility for communicating to patients the limits and extent of their medical care," writes Nicola E. Rubinow, a Hartford, Connecticut lawyer. "Health care providers should properly educate health care consumers about the nature of a particular condition, the probability of cure and the possibility of complication." [*San Francisco Chronicle-Examiner*. April 6, 1986.]

Doctors need an understanding and acceptance that they are not God and that when they cannot do more, they should not blame the patient or desert them. To the patient, death is not always an enemy, but rather a friend to be welcomed. It is no doubt necessary for anyone in the medical profession to keep some distance from the patient's struggle; however, if they are too aloof, then they become robots, less sensitive than mechanics repairing cars.

Doctors need to put more stress on areas of pain relief, especially for terminally ill patients, alleviating as much suffering as possible. A desire to achieve medical miracles should not take precedence over compassion for the patient and the family, or be attempted at their expense both in terms of suffering and finance.

David Hilfiker, M.D., author of *Healing the Wounds: A Physician Looks at His Work* wrote recently, "I still believe it is possible for patient and physician to share medical decision making, even in the most complex situation, but this cooperation requires a delicate blend of trust, time and a sensitivity that is too often lacking in the physician-patient relationship." [*Vogue*. November, 1986.]

Such cooperation, trust, time and sensitivity must be restored. It is a matter of life and death.

Hospitals

FOR A CONTINUOUS PERIOD of more than eleven years, I had a close member of my family in acute care hospitals, convalescent hospitals, or skilled nursing facilities located in the states of Nevada, California and Illinois. I have worked with doctors, nurses and staff in all of these, seeing to the care of loved ones.

I most firmly agree with Dr. Alan Robbins, chief of geriatrics at UCLA Medical Center, who has stated: "Going into the hospital for any reason is a very stressful experience for anybody. This factor is often seriously underestimated by health professionals." [*San Francisco Chronicle* August 27, 1984.]

To doctors and nurses, the hospital is simply where they work, their place of employment.

To the patient and the patient's family, it is a journey into the unknown at a time when pain, fear and uncertainty are the ruling emotions. Although a number of books have been written to prepare one for a hospital stay, few of us have the time or the opportunity for such advance planning. Both of Dan's hospital confinements in 1982 were emergency situations and he arrived in a completely helpless condition. To have to rely on someone else for every aspect of one's life is terrifying. Add to that our loss of control over where we will get our treatment and how long we will stay and we have a fearful combination.

Not so long ago, when people were ill they were admitted to the hospital where they stayed until they had recovered sufficiently to return home. Consideration was given to the individual home environment. If the doctor knew the patient lived alone, that there was no family close by or other help available, the patient stayed in the hospital until independent in self-care.

We no longer have "the hospital" and doctors are no longer allowed the privilege of always looking out for the best interests of their patients.

Now we have the acute care hospital, the convalescent hospital, both intermediate and board and care facilities, and, in some locales, hospice care and outpatient services. The length of stay in the acute care hospital and the convalescent hospital is strictly regulated in cost-containment moves by the government in Medicare and

Medicaid and by private insurance. These regulations spill over into the treatment that we all receive, regardless of age. Learning about these different facilities, making appropriate choices, securing the proper care for ourselves and our loved ones is a difficult and time-consuming task. The idea that the hospital is not a place for sick people to stay seems illogical, but it is one we have to face, as we also have to learn all the new vocabulary that has entered into the health care field.

A number of years ago, when I was studying life insurance law, I remember the admonition that it doesn't matter what type of legalese you may use in a policy provision, it is what the words mean to the man on the street that makes the words enforceable. As we were exposed to each new situation, Dan and I developed a sort of bizarre game, comparing our previous understanding of various terms with the current usage in the medical community. For example:

Layman's Understanding	Medical Definition
Hospital—a place for sick people	Acute care facility—a short term hotel, only for those people we can cure
Old folks' home	Convalescent hospital, skilled nursing facility, nursing home
Pain—suffering from which I want relief	An expected discomfort in the treatment of an illness
Discharge—fear, what next, where do I go, who will help me now	From the acute care facility—next patient, please
Dignity—being covered by a robe or sheet over my hospital gown, death without wires, tubes or unnecessary mutilation of my body	Not losing the battle to the disease

Death—fear of the un-	An unsatisfactory conclusion of
known, respite from pain	treatment
and suffering, home to	
my Father's arms	

Patients who are old enough for Medicare have to learn the meanings in the alphabet soup, such as DRG, PPS, and PRO. Most private insurances have similar rules.

DRG   (diagnostic-related group): the division of illnesses into related groups to determine the average costs of treatment

PPS   (prospective payment system): the Medicare hospital reimbursement system, which is a flat rate paid to the hospital for each patient based on the average cost of the diagnosis

UR   (utilization review): the hospital's internal review to determine the appropriate length of stay for each patient, conducted by a committee of health care professionals

PRO   (peer review organization): an organization established in every state, external to the hospital, to investigate complaints about patient treatment and to review both the quality and level of care necessary for the patient's treatment

But the phrase that strikes terror into us all is "premature discharge."

Near the end of Dan's first acute-care hospital confinement, there was a wide divergence of opinion among the doctor, nurses and therapists as to his condition. The nurses and therapists did not believe I could care for him by myself. The doctor set a discharge date and I know he was under pressure from the hospital to do so even though there was no question as to payment. We had excellent insurance but we were prepared to pay for any treatment our insurance did not cover. However, no one asked if we would or could pay for extra days if our insurance placed a limit. The automatic procedure was simply put into effect. Our physician knew nothing of our family situation and did not ask. When I told him there were just the two of us, he referred me to the discharge planner who was too busy to give me any time. I did not know what to expect or what we might need. The only provision made, *at* my request, was that a visiting nurse would come to see us in a few days. As Dan was somewhat mobile at this point and I was able to suspend most of my work to care for him, we managed.

During his second confinement, we had not thought of discharge, for we both assumed his time was so short that he would be spared another painful move. One day the discharge planner entered the room, without any warning, and stated she had a place for Dan at a local convalescent hospital, one we would not even consider. The Director of Nursing at the convalescent hospital of our choice worked with our doctor and Dan was able to stay in the acute care hospital a few extra days until there was an opening. We were fortunate. Still, he had to endure the physical agony of the move, being transported by ambulance for several miles, and the mental anguish of adjusting to a new environment at a time when he was in severe pain and awaiting the release of death.

Since then the rules are much stricter. My sister, who was eligible for Medicare, was not so fortunate following her December 1984 back surgery. When her "time was up" she was automatically transferred to a convalescent hospital. Her doctor assured her he would visit her there. Three days went by. No one checked her incision or changed her bandage. Her doctor did not come. She developed a fever. When my niece came to the hospital, she immediately called the doctor who readmitted my sister to the acute care facility. Additional surgery was performed to clean out the incision and to drain the staphylococcus infection which had developed. When my sister asked her doctor why he hadn't been to see her, he said he just couldn't go to convalescent hospitals. "It's too depressing."*

As it turned out, Dan's transfer to the convalescent hospital was a blessing. He left the acute care facility severely constipated, to the point of impaction.

His skin had broken down in two areas of painful, red splotches. These conditions were soon corrected. During the final five weeks of his life, he was cared for in a convalescent hospital that is highly regarded.

Entire books have been written on how to choose a convalescent hospital or nursing home. We had located this one in 1978 when we had moved his mother near us following her massive stroke. We visited all the convalescent hospitals in the area, not once but several

---

* California law requires that the physician see the patient within forty-eight hours after admission to a skilled nursing facility.

times. We went at mealtimes and noted the food, the help available to patients who could not feed themselves. We were aware of the cleanliness of the facility and of the staff. We went near the close of visiting hours and watched while patients were prepared for bed. We listened to the conversations and the noise level. We had found only one in which we had confidence. Even before Dan's confinement we had both spent many hours there with his mother.

A good convalescent hospital does a tremendous service. Their employees know and understand about death and care for their patients with gentleness, compassion and a depth of understanding. But Dan was twenty years younger than any other patient. As in all such hospitals, most of the patients were quite elderly. Many suffered from Alzheimer's, senility and mental confusion. Dan had a private room, removing him from such associations and I was with him during most of his waking hours; still, the atmosphere was depressing and he was kept awake by the shouters. The rooms were not especially attractive. It is more important to use limited funds on patient care than on cosmetic surroundings. Facilities are needed for care of patients who, like Dan, are young, vital, mentally alert, but who are dying.

During the past fifteen years, the home hospice movement has been growing rapidly. Home hospice groups are nonprofit organizations offering skilled and compassionate care to patients with life-threatening illness and to their families. Services may include nursing, home health aides, respite care, emotional support and counseling. In some areas there are hospice residential care facilities, but usually the hospice team works with families in the home to aid in patient care and family support. However, the extent of services available differs widely from one locale to another so it is necessary to determine what is available in your area and whether it would be appropriate given the condition of the patient and the family situation. The hospice movement claims to be more aware of pain and more involved in its control, yet studies reveal some controversy about this. I doubt that pain control is adequate under any setting due to the legal limitations put on the use of drugs.

We seriously considered home care but decided against it. A nurse friend asked me, "Mary, if Dan died at home, would you be able to continue living in your house?"

I don't know. If the family involved more than just Dan and me, perhaps. Then he would have been one presence among several. In a household of just two people, I'm really not sure if I could have returned to that house, that room, that bed.

We had no family close by for support. Today there are few old family homesteads with their spacious rooms where, in the past, nurses could have been hired to live in and be available for patient care twenty-four hours each day. I wasn't sure our small home would even accommodate a hospital bed and there were no extra rooms for live-in help, even if such help had been available.

Our insurance policy covered out-of-hospital care only for registered nurses and licensed practical nurses up to a limit of sixteen hours per day with a $5,000 overall maximum. We had previously paid $56 per hour for the visiting nurse, which was more than the daily charge for the convalescent hospital.

I had the responsibility for care of the home, the car, our finances, filling out endless forms . . . all the demands of daily life which do not stop because there is illness in the family. Care of the patient is added to these other responsibilities. But regardless of cost, whether covered by insurance or directly out of pocket, our primary concern was Dan's care. We both had doubts as to the reliability of volunteer caregivers. His condition and his pain made twenty-four hour care a necessity. What would we do if our helpers failed to show up? Once released from the hospital, the patient no longer has access to the same level of medical care, even though we wanted no expensive technology, just comfort.

Would I have the stamina to hold up under this round-the-clock responsibility? Would we be able to maintain any quality in our remaining days together under such circumstances?

Some of my friends who have attempted to work with hospice or home care have been disappointed and sometimes physically unable to continue. Then they have had difficulty in gaining admission for their loved ones into the convalescent hospital. When there is a shortage of rooms, priority is given to people being released from acute care facilities. Also, a patient must be hospitalized for at least three days prior to admittance to a skilled nursing facility in order to be covered by Medicare Part A.

Home care advocates insist that home care is less expensive, but not everyone agrees. Some researchers say that whether home care is less expensive depends on whether a person needs a range of services around-the-clock, which is costly, or merely a homemaker to clean and cook for a few hours.

Certainly all types of care must be considered, but the decisions must be personal. Some families have stalwart sons who can move or turn the patient. Some wives are especially good at nursing the sick. Some have extended families and relatives available to help to relieve the burden. What works for one family will not work for another. It is necessary to take cognizance of individual strengths and weaknesses. There is no *one* right way. Just as the patient does not "fail" simply because he cannot get well, neither does the family "fail" when they require help. Each of us must disregard the pressures of others—family, friends, doctors—and make the decision we can best live with, the one which will be based upon the welfare and peace of mind of the patient and will provide him/her quality of life during the last days. Each should be allowed to do this without any sense of guilt, yet the current trend is to treat all patients and all families the same.

That proper hospital care is an urgent problem is evidenced by the many newspaper and magazine articles on the subject. We read of people being released quicker and sicker, of patient-dumping, of patients put at risk by transfers.

George J. Annas, associate professor of law and medicine at Boston University, says that "each patient should have access to a person whose job it is to work for the patient to help the patient exercise the patient's rights, and who has the authority to obtain medical records, medical consultations, delay discharge, question medical and nursing care, and lodge complaints directly with the chief of staff, administrator and board of trustees without fear of retaliation."[*San Francisco Chronicle*. June 19, 1982.]

Some hospitals do have patient's advocates. Although the job title may read "patient's advocate," they are still hospital employees.

During my sister's confinement in the spring of 1986, her roommate was a 90-year old woman with a broken hip. She said it was the first time she had ever been in a hospital. The day following her surgery, while she was still groggy from the medication, I watched as a hospital employee less than half her age came into the room and explained that she could only stay in the acute care hospital number of days. Then they would have to send her to the convalescent hospital where she would be permitted to spend ___ days, and then she would have to go home. (She lived by herself in an apartment.)

I bit my tongue to keep from lashing out at this insensitivity. Do we want a health care delivery system that, the first day you are in the hospital, has someone at your bedside telling you when and where you have to go?

The National Committee to Preserve Social Security and Medicare has printed a "Medicare Patient's Bill of Rights" on a wallet-sized card, as follows:

Medicare Patient Bill of Rights

1. Right to proper care—Your discharge date should be determined solely by your medical needs, not by Medicare payments.
2. Right to information—The hospital must inform you about decisions affecting your Medicare coverage or the length of your stay.
3. Right to Appeal—If the hospital wants to discharge you too soon, appeal the decision to the Federal Peer Review Organization (PRO). You cannot be dismissed pending your appeal.

How to Appeal a Hospital Discharge

If you are told that Medicare will no longer pay for your hospital stay:

1. Demand a written notice of explanation from the hospital immediately. The PRO will need this written notice to review your appeal.
2. Call or write the PRO. You can get the number and address of your local PRO from your hospital or by calling your local Social Security office. Your appeal can take up to three working days, and you may have to pay for additional hospital costs if you lose your appeal.

The state of California requires that a patient's bill of rights and a consent for treatment be given to each patient upon admission to a skilled nursing facility. The patients and their families can review their financial records at the hospital whenever they request to do so.

It has been my experience that the quality of care at such facilities does fluctuate, usually because of staffing problems. Any complaints about patient care can be lodged with the Department of Health Services, who will then investigate. Strict confidentiality is observed. The Department of Health Services does annual reviews of each facility and the records of inspection are open to the public.

Local Councils on Aging can be of assistance, or you can contact the National Center for State Long-term Care Ombudsman Resources, 2033 K Street N.W., Suite 304, Washington, D.C. 20006.

But what of patients without families who are too ill to protest? And those of us who are too young to be involved in the Medicare system? The rules are tightened each day and I, like millions of people alone, worry about who will be my advocate when it is my turn.

Dr. Fazlur Rahman, chief of hematology and oncology at Angelo Community Hospital in San Angelo, Texas, wrote: "As a cancer specialist, I often see patients who are not candidates for chemotherapy, radiation treatment or surgery but nonetheless need hospital care for distressing complications. They cannot be taken care of by home health-care services, hospices or nursing homes. Not treating cancer is one thing, not treating a person is another." [*San Francisco Chronicle*. January 15, 1986.]

Doctors are quoted as fearing a tug-of-war between what is medically best for their patient and what is financially prudent for the hospital. To the patient, this struggle may mean life or death.

"In the rush created by doctors, lawyers and insurance companies to protect their interests, protections for health-care consumers sometimes receive inadequate attention," stated Doris Reeves Lipscomb, deputy director of state legislation for American Association of Retired Persons. [*Modern Maturity*. April/May, 1986.]

Read "consumer" as "patient," meaning you or your loved one, and see the difference in impact.

Jack Owen, Washington representative of the American Hospital Association, said that shorter hospital stays don't necessarily mean lower charges because "as you lower the length of stay the fixed costs don't change." [*The Press Democrat*. December 3, 1986.]

Dr. William B. Schwartz, professor of medicine at Tufts University School of Medicine and a leading economist, explains that "the primary culprits in rising hospital costs are rapidly advancing technology, the labor-intensive character of hospital care and a growing population—none of which is appreciably affected by the current cost-containment efforts." [*Senior Spectrum*. February, 1987.]

Yet we continue to read of patients being released in delicate conditions, even as hospitals rush to buy nursing homes and to try to attract new "clients" by spending money on redecoration, fresh flowers in rooms and wine with meals.

Why couldn't the money be spent on keeping sick people in the hospital until they are able to go home, to improve service, training and treatment? Why can't the facilities already in place be better utilized? Why can't a wing or unused area of a hospital with its empty beds be converted to convalescent care or hospice care? It is easier on the patient to be wheeled down the hall than transferred by ambulance to another facility miles away, and the patient would have the assurance that comprehensive medical care was within reach.

What can we do?

We are advised to take a more active role; we are told that it is the responsibility of the patient to seek out and to insist upon the best medical care. We are advised that we must learn our rights. This theme is repeated regularly in newspaper and magazine articles. Several books have been written to help one prepare for a hospital confinement and, if time permits, these should be studied.

Charles P. Weikel, former Director of the western region of the U. S. Administration on Aging, recommends the free booklet, *Knowing Your Rights*, published by the American Association of Retired Persons. He also states that the patient should have assistance from a friend or relative who could make inquiries on the patient's behalf while in the hospital. The patient should also furnish the doctor and friend with written instructions as to his/her desires regarding the extent of treatment. [*Senior Spectrum*. March, 1987.]

A recent publication printed a *Homecare Checklist: What to Look For*, twenty-three items to be evaluated in choosing home care services for patients.

Is all this preparation realistic? Many confinements will be of emergency status and such advance planning will not be possible. People lead busy lives with full-time jobs, homes to care for, aging parents and/or children for whom they are responsible. This does not allow sufficient time to do exhaustive research on doctors, hospitals or a particular illness. Working people don't have time. Frail elderly don't have the ability. The rule of *caveat emptor*, "let the buyer beware," is not appropriate to health care. At some point, we have to trust the system.

Each one of us, however, can talk with our own doctor, explaining our fears and concerns. We must find a physician who is sympathetic with our quest for proper medical care and who will cooperate with us in getting it.

Since the problems of hospital care are rooted in costs, those of us who have the time and a particular interest in these problems must get more involved. We must voice our opinions and concerns to our representatives in local, state and federal government by cards, letters and phone calls. According to *Internal Medicine News*, "Free emergency and primary medical care are provided for members of Congress and their staffs. The Office of the Physician of Congress was established in 1928 and now has three physicians, eleven nurses, a pharmacy and administrative staff." Nevertheless, these are the people who pass the legislation on Medicare and Medicaid and whose decisions ultimately affect us all. [*The Press Democrat*. February 10, 1987.]

If health care dollars are finite, we will want to have our say about how they are spent.

"Researchers say that the public is responsible for rising health care costs as people acquire illnesses that cannot be cured easily or cheaply." [*The New Yorker*. October 15, 1984.]

Statistics show that 60 to 70 percent of Americans spend the most money on health care in the last six months of life.

Do these statements surprise anyone?

We don't go to the doctor unless we are ill, and in our later years we frequently have illnesses which lead to death; however, the funds spent in the last few months of life could be reduced if life support systems were not so widely used.

Though artificial hearts may be more interesting, if we have to make a choice, do we want to pay for bionic people or for pain relief?

Will dollars go to couples who want children and therefore finance test-tube babies and embryo transplants, or to patients suffering from cancer, diabetes, arthritis, osteoporosis, Alzheimer's disease?

One heart-lung transplant costs more than most families spend on medical care in a lifetime. Do we want the dangerous and dubiously successful procedures which drain dollars from forms of care whose benefits are already known?

Are all funds to be spent on technology or will some be used for prevention?

Is medical care to be available only to the very rich, or those with excellent cost-effective insurance coverage?

These are concerns which affect us all and we need to express our views to the people who make the rules. Organ transplants and test-tube conceptions are now being covered by some insurance companies. This translates to higher premiums for us all. We must decide what we, the patients (consumers) are willing to pay for and let our insurance companies, unions, federal, state and local officials know our desires.

We can support organizations, such as the American Association of Retired Persons, which is working to help protect patients' rights under Medicare and Medicaid.

We can write articles for local papers and letters to the editors.

We can visit our local hospitals and convalescent hospitals, perhaps do volunteer work there, observe and report any abuses that we see. There is a Medicare Peer Review Organization in every state. We can give support to our friends and relatives who are patients.

We can work with organizations such as the County Council on Aging or County Commission on Senior Care. We will all eventually reach that age.

We can suggest programs on the various aspects of health care and cost containment to our local service organizations: Rotary, Kiwanis, Soroptimist. Get people interested.

I frequently receive brochures through the mail from the Cancer Society, the Heart Association, the local junior college, hospital ministries association, or some other organization announcing a seminar on health care and health decisions and I attend as many of these as I can. I want to keep informed.

I joined the California Health Decisions-North Bay, an organization to foster community dialogue about the ethical, financial and legal dilemmas in health care and attended some of their workshops to get the layman's input on such matters as access to health care, individual rights, prevention, quality and allocation. Some of the questions discussed were:

- Do people have the right to health care? How much?
- What categories should take priority?
- How and by whom should resources be allotted?
- Are we obliged to prolong life by every means? When should we stop? Who decides?

I want to have my say in answering these questions. I want to have some effect on the decision-making process. If doctors are caught between patient and hospital, how will the patient fare? Will the quality of care suffer? I believe it already has. We must work to change that. We must keep the heart in medicine.

PATIENT'S RIGHTS

Skilled Nursing Facilities
Intermediate Care Facilities

All patients shall have rights which include, but are not limited to the following: The right

(1) To be fully informed, as evidenced by the patient's written acknowledgement prior to or at the time of admission and during stay, of these rights and of all rules and regulations governing patient conduct.

(2) To be fully informed, prior to or at the time of admission and during stay, of services available in the facility and of related charges, including any charges for services not covered by the facility's basic per diem rate or not covered under Titles XVIII or XIX of the Social Security Act.

(3) To be fully informed by a physician of his or her medical condition, unless medically contraindicated, and to be afforded the opportunity to participate in the planning of medical treatment and to refuse to participate in experimental research.

(4) To refuse treatment to the extent permitted by law and to be informed of the medical consequences of such refusal.

(5) To be transferred or discharged only for medical reasons, or the patient's welfare or that of other patients or for nonpayment for his or her stay and to be given reasonable advance notice to ensure orderly transfer or discharge. Such actions shall be documented in the patient's health record.

(6) To be encouraged and assisted throughout the period of stay to exercise his or her rights as a patient and as a citizen, and to this end to voice grievances and recommend changes in policies and services to facility staff and/or outside representatives of the patient's choice, free from restraint, interference, coercion, discrimination or reprisal.

(7) To manage his or her personal financial affairs or to be given at least a quarterly accounting of financial transactions made on the patient's behalf should the facility accept his or her written delegation of this responsibility.

(8) To be free from mental and physical abuse and to be free from chemical and (except in emergencies) physical restraints except

as authorized in writing by a physician or other person lawfully authorized to prescribe care for a specified and limited period of time, or when necessary to protect the patient from injury to themselves or to others.

(9) To be assured confidential treatment of his or her personal and medical records and to approve or refuse their release to any individual outside the facility, except in the case of his or her transfer to another health facility, or as required by law or third party payment contract.

(10) To be treated with consideration, respect and full recognition of the patient's dignity and individuality, including privacy in treatment and in care of the patient's personal needs.

(11) Not to be required to perform services for the facility that are not included for therapeutic purposes in the patient's plan of care.

(12) To associate and communicate privately with persons of the patient's choice, and to send and receive his or her personal mail unopened, unless medically contraindicated.

(13) To meet with others and participate in activities of social, religious, and community groups, unless medically contraindicated.

(14) To retain and use his or her personal clothing and possessions as space permits, unless to do so would infringe upon the rights of other patients and unless medically contraindicated.

(15) If married, to be assured privacy for visits by the patient's spouse and if both are patients in the facility, to be permitted to share a room, unless medically contraindicated.

(16) To have daily visiting hours established.

(17) To have visits from members of the clergy at any time at the request of the patient or the patient's guardian.

(18) To allow relatives, or persons responsible, to visit critically ill patients at any time unless medically contraindicated.

(19) To be allowed privacy for visits with family, friends, clergy, social workers or for professional or business purposes.

(20) To have reasonable access to telephones to make and receive confidential calls.

(21) To be permitted to purchase drugs or rent or purchase medical supplies or equipment.

Preplanning

WRITER ERIC LAX, author of *Life & Death on 10 West*, a study of life in a cancer ward at UCLA Medical Center, was quoted as saying, "When you're on that ward, there's no life outside. It's such a gripping environment that you forget your responsibility as a functioning person elsewhere." And he was just an observer.

How much more difficult it is for the patient and the patient's family to cope with the demands of the outside world at this traumatic time, yet the world does continue to make its demands and to intrude into the sickroom. Bills must be paid. Insurance forms must be completed. Taxes must be figured and filed. Decisions must be made. All the tedium of daily life goes on even as one is involved in the life and death struggle. In our situation, we had not only our own affairs to take care of, but Dan's mother's as well. Now this fell entirely to me. I could not devote all my time and energy to the sickroom. Advance planning helped to alleviate the burdens.

While there is some question as to the need for, indeed, the advisability of, the annual physical examination, there is no doubt of the benefits of the annual financial checkup. Early in our marriage we started the habit of listing assets and liabilities at the end of each year and of determining our net worth. Such figures, however, are only a beginning.

An adequate annual statement includes information on the following:

1. Assets, liabilities & net worth
2. Insurance coverage, group
3. Insurance coverage, private
4. Social Security benefits
5. Retirement benefits/pension plans
6. Will
7. Power of Attorney
8. Durable Power of Attorney for Health Care
9. Funeral Plans
10. Miscellaneous

Assets & Liabilities & Net Worth

This is the starting point. With the emotional, physical and mental stress of illness, there comes the financial cost which must be confronted. A statement of net worth will reassure you as to the resources which you have available.

1. List the names & addresses of banks, saving & loans, credit unions and all financial institutions where accounts are maintained and the amounts in each.
2. Real estate: Show location, value, name and address of lien holder, if any.
3. List other assets.
4. List names and addresses of all persons or institutions to whom money is owed and the amounts.
5. Subtract total liabilities from total assets to determine net worth.

Insurance, Group

Review all fringe benefits available from your place of employment, including any paid sick leave. Determine what you can expect in the event of the disability or death of the breadwinner.

Dan's employer furnished a statement each year of various fringe benefits, and with my training in insurance I was able to calculate any figures not quoted. This information should, however, be available from your employer's personnel department.

1. Medical insurance coverage
2. Disability benefits, amount and length of period payable
3. Life insurance, amounts, names of beneficiaries.

Look for gaps in coverages and limitations or conditions to be met. For example, Dan's disability income benefits increased each year, based upon his annual salary; however, the increase was contingent upon his being actively at work on the first working day of January. Since his last day of work was December 16, his disability income would have been $200 less per month than we anticipated. Medical insurance has some surprising limits on home care and convalescent hospital coverage, though some liberalization is in process. Consider the purchase of additional insurance to fill these gaps.

Insurance, Private

For each company in which you hold insurance, list the following:

1. Name and address of insurance company
2. Name, address and phone number of servicing agent
3. Policy number and name of insured
4. Name of beneficiary

Do you need to make any changes in the beneficiary designations? Circumstances and needs change. We had originally designated our mothers as secondary beneficiaries in our life insurance policies. When they both became unable to take care of their own affairs through a combination of age and illness, we removed their names and designated Dan's brother and my sister, who would be responsible for their care and their finances.

My aunt recently passed away at age 87. Her parents were still listed on the life insurance policy she had purchased in 1932.

Do *not* store policies in your safe-deposit box where they might not be readily available at time of need, but instead, keep them in a safe place at home.

When it becomes necessary to contact any insurance carrier, remember to make a note of the name and title of the person you contact. Though applications for group insurance benefits will usually be handled through your employer's personnel department, the rules for handling any claims for both private and group insurance are the same. When submitting claim forms and correspondence, always keep a photocopy for your own records. Also, make and keep copies of any doctors' bills, hospital bills, or other charges which you are submitting either for payment or for reimbursement.

Social Security

For most of us, Social Security is the basis of not only retirement, but also disability benefits, and it is of the utmost importance that we keep a list of Social Security numbers of all covered persons in the family readily available. As employees, we should also keep copies of our W-2 forms, Wage and Tax Statement, showing yearly Social Security contributions and should periodically request from Social Security a Summary Statement of Earnings to see if all contributions have been properly credited to our account.

Current estimates of benefits payable in the event of disability, retirement or death are available from Social Security offices. Private insurance agents can also provide estimates of these. Since benefits frequently change, it is well to pick up pamphlets from the office and review them from time to time.

As with private insurance, when contact is made with anyone in the Social Security Administration, be sure to get their name and title and keep a copy of all papers filed.

Retirement Benefits/Pension Plans

While not part of the information you normally think of at time of illness, these figures should be included in any annual financial statement. In the event a disability should continue until retirement age (usually anytime from age 55 on), the monthly retirement benefits could then become part of your financial security.

Will

Unless one is content with having the state dispose of his assets and property for him, serious consideration must be given to who gets what at the time of death. The usual method of transferring properties is through a will.

One of the more stressful times during Dan's illness came when we suddenly remembered our wills and discovered they were out of date. We had not given them a thought since they were first made. When we had made the changes in our insurance beneficiaries, we had overlooked the wills. We needed to change these too. There had also been some changes made in the tax laws that affected us. To have to make the changes at a time when Dan was in the hospital struggling to get well was emotionally upsetting.

Family situations do change, both as to need and as to

circumstances. Tax laws are revised. Federal and state inheritance laws are updated.* A will must be a living document that is reviewed regularly to be certain it meets current needs, or reflects current desires.

There are, however, other means for settling estates and avoiding probate, among them the revocable living trust and joint tenancy which carries with it a right of survivorship. Since every individual case and each family situation is unique, such decisions should be made only after adequate counsel by a qualified attorney (preferably one who specializes in estate matters), a financial counselor and tax consultant.

But whatever method of disposal of an estate is selected, it must be reviewed regularly and not just filed away, out of sight and out of mind.

This is also a good time to prepare a letter of instructions for your executor, who will need to know the following:

- Location of your will, birth certificate, marriage certificate, service discharge, and other important papers and keys.
- Name of your attorney.
- Names and addresses of heirs.
- Location of records, such as tax return copies.
- Names of financial institutions in which you have accounts and/or safe deposit boxes.
- List of contents of safe deposit box.
- Insurance companies, policy numbers, and location of policies.
- Your Social Security number.
- Location and description of any real estate owned.
- Location of burial plot and any funeral plans.
- Any other special instructions which would be needed to carry out executor duties.

This information can be in the form of a letter which is sealed to be opened only in the event of death. A copy should also be

---

* The federal estate tax exemption was increased to $600,000 in 1987. At present, assets left to a surviving spouse are exempt from federal estate tax. State inheritance tax rules vary widely.

furnished to a member of your family. I have prepared such a letter and sent copies to my executor, my niece, and my brother-in-law to be opened in the event of my death or disability.

Power of Attorney

Dan's mother was mentally alert but incapacitated from the effects of her stroke. He was able to take charge of her business through a Power of Attorney. I have now completed such a form.

Would someone be able to step in to take care of your business if you were unable to? Consider signing a Power of Attorney to someone you trust to make decisions for you if you are incapable of making them for yourself.

Durable Power of Attorney for Health Care

Dr. Benjamin Spock has been quoted as saying, "I don't fear the dying as long as it's not very painful or lonely or lacking in dignity." [*Parade.* March 10, 1985.]

Yet modern medical technology can keep many terminal patients alive indeterminately. Therefore, we must, at some time, make a decision as to what action we wish taken in the event we are struck with a devastating illness. Do we want the medical community to do everything possible to prolong life, using all heroics and life-support systems available, or do we, like Dr. Spock, wish to die with as much dignity and comfort as possible? We should make this decision instead of leaving it in the hands of family and physician, or risking untold suffering by being kept alive against our wishes.

Dan was mentally and physically able to make his decision and to communicate it at the time when he wanted treatment discontinued. His body was wasting away. He was in constant pain, partially paralyzed and bedridden. What if his mind had been active but he was unable to communicate? *I* knew what his desires were, but would my instructions have been honored? What about those of us who have no family, or at least none close by?

Since his death, California has approved the Durable Power of Attorney for Health Care so that I now have the privilege of making my personal decision and informing my doctor of that decision.

DIRECTIVE TO PHYSICIANS

Directive made this _____ day of _____(month, year).

I _____, being of sound mind, willfully and voluntarily make known my desire that my life shall not be artificially prolonged under the circumstances set forth below, do hereby declare:

1. If at any time I should have an incurable injury, disease, or illness certified to be a terminal condition by two physicians, and where the application of life-sustaining procedures would serve only to artificially prolong the moment of my death and where my physician determines that my death is imminent whether or not life-sustaining procedures are utilized, I direct that such procedures be withheld or withdrawn, and that I be permitted to die naturally.

2. In the absence of my ability to give directions regarding the use of such life-sustaining procedures, it is my intention that this directive shall be honored by my family and physician(s) as the final expression of my legal right to refuse medical or surgical treatment and accept the consequences from such refusal.

3. If I have been diagnosed as pregnant and that diagnosis is known to my physician, this directive shall have no force or effect during the course of my pregnancy.

4. I have been diagnosed at least 14 days ago as having a terminal condition by _____M.D., whose address is _____, and whose telephone number is _____. I understand that if I have not filled in the physician's name and address, it shall be presumed that I did not have a terminal condition when I made out this directive.

5. This directive shall have no force or effect five years from the date filled in above.

6. I understand the full import of this directive and I am emotionally and mentally competent to make this directive.

Signed_____

City, County and State of Residence_____

The declarant has been personally known to me and I believe him or her to be of sound mind.

Witness_____   Witness_____

I have also given my niece the power to make such health care decisions for me in the event I am not able. This is the best I can do to guarantee that my wishes will be honored.

Several states have passed "living will" legislation allowing people to sign legally binding instructions to stop treatment and disconnect life-support systems when death is imminent and damage is irreversible. Living Will forms are available from the Society for the Right to Die, 250 West 57th St., New York, NY 10107. This organization also publishes newsletters which keep members informed as to legislation pending in various states to permit withdrawal of life-support systems and allowing death with dignity.

Organ Transplants

There is another important decision to be made and communicated. Even before death, family members may be asked by the hospital staff what the patient's desires are on the controversial and highly personal subject of organ transplants. This is a decision best made by the patient and so indicated before the occasion arises rather than as a callous intrusion into personal grief. The State of California has a place on the driver's license form for you to indicate if you wish to have any usable organs donated at the time of your death. A brochure has been prepared and distributed through the Boy Scouts of America on the donor awareness program and includes a donor card to be completed and registered with the American Council on Transplantation in Washington, DC. The instructions can be general or specific. Since this decision must be made eventually, it is best made at a more rational time than at the deathbed.

Funeral Plans

While this is not a subject of importance to all persons, some of us feel very strongly about what we want done at the time of our death, and the only way we can hope that our wishes will be carried out is to be sure they are known. Dan had completed his Masonic lodge book indicating his preference in funeral arrangements and we had purchased our burial plots some years before. Funeral plans should include:

1. Location of burial plot, if already purchased. If not, consider such a purchase.
2. Names and addresses of persons to be notified.
3. Preferred mortuary. It is possible to make all funeral arrangements at the mortuary and pay for them in advance.
4. Type of service.
5. Disposition of remains.

While my sister was still mobile, she and I went to the local mortuary in our hometown and made complete funeral arrangements for our mother, our aunt, and for Bobby herself. We selected the caskets and the vaults, designated the ministers to perform the services, arranged for the music, and we prepaid all this by setting up trust accounts with the funeral home. Family plots in the local cemetery had previously been purchased. This gave Bobby great satisfaction and peace of mind during her last year. And since these three loved ones died within a period of less than thirteen months, this advance planning was of immeasurable help to me. I knew that I was carrying out their wishes. I have prepared all of this same information for myself in a letter of instructions, including favorite passages of scripture and favorite hymns.

Miscellaneous

Assemble birth certificates, marriage certificates, death certificates, military service discharge papers and keep them in a safe but accessible place.

Make an inventory of the contents of your safe-deposit box and keep one list in the box and a duplicate list in a safe place at home.

Prepare a list of names, addresses and phone numbers of your attorney, executor and principal heirs. As a convenience, I keep a framed list by my telephone of the numbers of my doctor, dentist, lawyer, executor, closest relatives and friends, and the funeral parlor to which I wish to be taken.

With our educational backgrounds and our careers in insurance, Dan and I were probably more aware than most of the need for all these plans, yet we had not fully thought out the consequences of a life-threatening illness.

This annual update provides a perfect opportunity for meaningful discussion not only of financial affairs but also of affairs of a more personal nature. How does one want to be remembered? Which memories, beliefs and philosophies do we cling to and want preserved? Where would we want memorial contributions to go? Each day we live, we are creating history and making memories. Perhaps it is time to identify those boxes of snapshots and put them into albums, or maybe it is time to make a new memory. The photo albums of yesterday have become the videotapes of today, but regardless of how preserved, family memories are irreplaceable assets of any estate.

Dan's friends were pleased to receive an item of his jewelry. While not all of one's possessions are of sufficient value to be included in the formal Will, there may well be some preferences to be indicated.

Thoughts of this nature just naturally follow a study of what one has accumulated, where one has been, and where one is going, and they are healthy thoughts that help to put our priorities in order.

Is such planning morbid?

I don't think so. It is a comfort to the patient to know that all possible has been done to provide for loved ones. It is equally reassuring to those loved ones to know that they have carried out the wishes of the patient.

As we were returning from Aunt Helen's funeral, my great-niece Sue turned to me and said, "Aunt Mary, God forbid that anything should happen to you, but do you have all your plans made?"

I assured her that I did. Now we can all get on with the business of living.

Recommended Reading

The following publications are free to AARP members and are available from AARP (American Association of Retired Persons), 1909 K St. N.W., Washington, DC 20049:

Checklist of Concerns, Resources for Caregivers

A Handbook About Care in the Home

Knowing Your Rights

Making Wise Decisions for Long-term Care

On Being Alone: A Guide for Widowed Persons

The following booklets are available from the Office of Cancer Communication, National Cancer Institute, Building 31, Room 10A24, Bethesda, MD 20892 (1-800-422-6237—hot line for patients):

Taking Time, Support for People with Cancer and the People Who Care About Them

Chemotherapy and You, A Guide to Self-help During Treatment

Radiation Therapy and You, A Guide to Self-help During Treatment

Eating Hints, Recipes and Tips for Better Nutrition During Cancer Treatment

These books may be helpful:

Caretaker's Manual, available from local American Cancer Society units.

Choosing a Nursing Home: A Guidebook for Families, by Marty Richards, University of Washington Press, Seattle, 1985.

I'll Never Walk Alone: The Inspiring Story of a Teenager's Struggle Against Cancer, by Carol Simonides, as told to Diane Gage. Continuum, New York, 1983.

Let the Patient Decide, by Louis Shattuck Baer, M.D. The Westminster Press, Philadelphia, 1978.

Medical Care Can Be Dangerous to Your Health, by Eugene D. Robin, M.D. Harper & Row, New York, 1986.

A Physician Faces Cancer in Himself, by Samuel Sanes, M.D. State University of New York Press, Albany, NY, 1979.

Prescription Drugs and Their Side Effects, by Edward L. Stern. Grosset & Dunlap, New York, 1981.

Public Affairs Pamphlets No. 515, *Drugs—Use, Misuse, Abuse Guidance for Families*, and No. 570, *Know Your Medication*. 381 Park Ave. South, New York, NY, 10016.

A Second Start: A Widow's Guide to Financial Survival at a Time of Emotional Crisis, by Judith N. Brown, L.L.B., and Christina Baldwin. Simon & Shuster, New York, 1986.

When Bad Things Happen to Good People, by Harold S. Kushner. Schocken Books, New York, 1981.

You Can Take It With You: Estate Planning, by Edwin C. Anderson. Redwood City, CA. David S. Lake Publishers, 1981.

Books to help you prepare for a hospital stay:

The People's Hospital Book, by Dr. Ronald Gots and Dr. Arthur Kaufman. Avon, 1981

The Hospital Experience, by Judith Nierenberg and Florence Janovic. Berkley, 1985

Take This Book to the Hospital With You, by Charles B. Inlander and Ed Weiner. Rodale, 1985

So You're Having an Operation: A Step-by-Step Guide to Controlling Your Hospital Stay, by Karen R. Williams and Janet Stensaas. Prentice Hall, 1985